MELANOMA
DIET COOKBOOK FOR BEGINNERS

Delicious Recipes and Vital Nutritional Guidance for Healing, Wellness, and Recovery

Kingsley Klopp

To show our appreciation for your purchase, we're delighted to offer you these special bonuses as a heartfelt thank you.

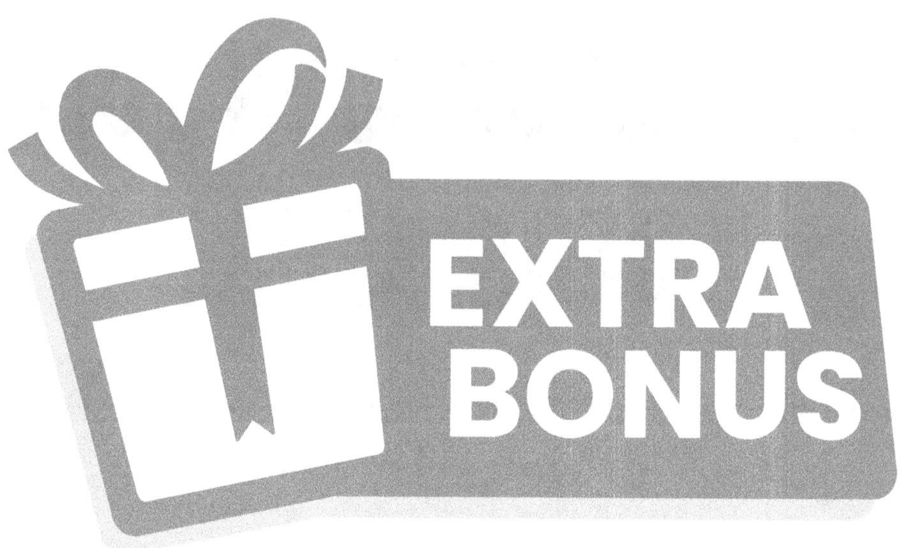

1. A Food Tracker Journal
2. Downloadable E-BOOK featuring full-color images of finished recipes

Table of Content

Important Note

We're thrilled to accompany you on your journey towards better health and delicious eating. As you dive into these recipes, we want to share an important note to ensure your experience is both enjoyable and beneficial.

Individual Needs and Adjustments

Every person's body is unique, and dietary needs can vary widely from one individual to another. While the recipes in this cookbook are designed with general nutritional benefits in mind, it's crucial to remember that they might not be perfectly suited for everyone. Your health, treatment plan, and personal preferences are key factors in determining what works best for you. We encourage you to adjust these recipes based on your specific needs and tastes. Feel free to tweak ingredient quantities, substitute items, or make any modifications that suit your health and palate. Your comfort and satisfaction are our top priorities.

Consult with Your Healthcare Provider

Navigating dietary choices during a melanoma journey can sometimes be overwhelming. If you find yourself uncertain about certain ingredients or meal plans, we strongly recommend consulting with your healthcare provider. Your doctor, nutritionist, or dietitian can offer personalized advice that aligns with your medical needs and overall treatment plan.

Nutritional Information Disclaimer

Please note that the nutritional information provided for each recipe is approximate. Variations in ingredient brands, preparation methods, and portion sizes can influence the final nutritional content of your meals. We've done our best to provide accurate estimates, but these should be used as a general guide rather than an absolute measure.

Our Commitment to You

Our goal is to support you with recipes that nourish your body and delight your taste buds. We've poured love and care into crafting meals that are both nutritious and flavorful, designed to make your journey a little bit easier and a lot more delicious.

If our cookbook has brought joy to your kitchen and table, we'd be thrilled to hear about your experiences in an Amazon review. On the flip side, if you stumble upon any hiccups while exploring our recipes, don't hesitate to get in touch at **kloppkingsley@gmail.com.** We're here to support your cooking journey every step of the way.

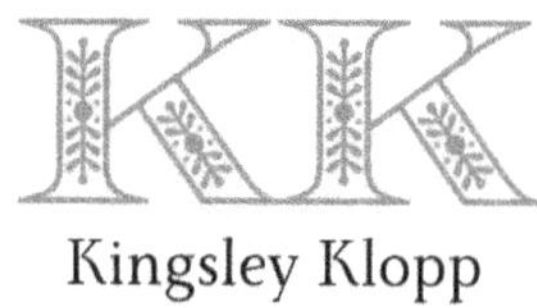

Kingsley Klopp

Introduction

Welcome to the **Melanoma Diet Cookbook for Beginners!** Whether you've recently been diagnosed with melanoma, are undergoing treatment, or are looking to support a loved one through this journey, you've picked up this book for one simple reason: food. Yes, the meals we share, the nourishment we take in, and the culinary joy we experience can make a significant difference in our lives, especially during challenging times. Food has always been more than just sustenance. It's a powerful tool for healing, a comfort in times of need, and a delightful journey of flavors that brings people together. In the face of melanoma, one of the most serious forms of skin cancer, the role of nutrition becomes even more critical. But before you picture bland hospital food or a life devoid of your favorite treats, let me reassure you: the recipes in this book are anything but boring. We're talking vibrant, flavorful dishes that will make your taste buds dance and your body thank you.

You might be wondering, *"How can a diet impact melanoma?"* Great question! While no food can cure cancer, a well-balanced diet can significantly bolster your body's natural defenses, help manage symptoms, and improve your overall well-being. Think of it as giving your body the best possible fuel to fight the good fight. In this book, you'll discover a variety of recipes rich in antioxidants, vitamins, and minerals, all designed to support your immune system, enhance your energy levels, and keep your spirits high. The journey of a thousand miles begins with a single step, and your journey towards better health and wellness starts right here. The "Melanoma Diet Cookbook for Beginners" isn't just about recipes; it's about embracing a lifestyle that promotes healing and vitality. We understand that the word "diet" can sometimes feel restrictive, but we're here to redefine that perception. This isn't about cutting out everything you love; it's about discovering new favorites and finding joy in the process. Our approach is simple yet effective: focus on fresh, whole foods that nourish your body from the inside out. We've packed this cookbook with easy-to-follow recipes that use accessible ingredients, ensuring you can whip up a nutritious meal without added stress. From hearty breakfasts that kickstart your day to comforting dinners that wrap up your evenings with a warm hug, we've got you covered.

Let's talk about some of the star players in our recipes. You'll find an abundance of leafy greens, berries, nuts, seeds, and lean proteins, each chosen for their health-boosting properties. These ingredients are not just good for you; they're incredibly versatile, lending themselves to a myriad of delicious dishes. Imagine starting your day with a refreshing berry smoothie bowl, snacking on crunchy kale chips in the afternoon, and savoring a flavorful quinoa salad for dinner. Sounds good, right?

But we're not stopping at nutrition alone. We're also going to delve into the emotional and psychological benefits of cooking and sharing meals. Food has the power to lift our spirits, bring us together, and create lasting memories. When you're facing a health challenge like melanoma, these moments of joy and connection become even more important. We'll provide tips on mindful eating, creating a positive dining environment, and even involving family and friends in your culinary journey. In addition to mouthwatering recipes, you'll find practical advice on meal planning, grocery shopping, and kitchen essentials. We know that life can be hectic, and the last thing you need is added complexity. That's why we've designed this cookbook to be as user-friendly as possible, making it easy for you to incorporate these healthy habits into your daily routine. To make your journey even smoother, we've included a chapter dedicated to understanding melanoma and the science behind the recommended dietary choices. Knowledge is power, and we want you to feel empowered to make informed decisions about your health. We'll break down the latest research in a way that's easy to understand, so you can feel confident in the choices you're making.

As you flip through these pages, let yourself be inspired by the vibrant colors, tantalizing aromas, and rich flavors that await you. Remember, this is more than just a cookbook; it's a companion on your path to wellness. Each recipe is a step towards a healthier, happier you, and we're honored to be part of your journey. So, grab your apron, roll up your sleeves, and let's get cooking. Here's to delicious meals, joyful moments, and a healthier tomorrow. Welcome to the **Melanoma Diet Cookbook for Beginners** – where every bite is a step towards healing.

Understanding Melanoma

What is Melanoma?.

What is Melanoma?

Melanoma is a type of skin cancer that originates in the melanocytes. These are the cells responsible for producing melanin, the pigment that gives our skin, hair, and eyes their color. When melanocytes begin to grow uncontrollably, they form a tumor, which we call melanoma.

Origins of Melanoma

To truly understand melanoma, we need to start at the cellular level. Melanocytes are located in the bottom layer of the epidermis, the outermost layer of our skin. They are critical in protecting our skin from harmful UV radiation by producing melanin, which absorbs and dissipates the UV rays.

However, when these cells are damaged, typically by excessive UV exposure from the sun or tanning beds, their DNA can mutate. These mutations can cause the melanocytes to grow uncontrollably, leading to the development of melanoma.

Development and Progression of Melanoma

Melanoma can develop anywhere on the skin but is most common in areas that receive significant sun exposure, such as the back, legs, arms, and face. However, it can also occur in less exposed areas like the soles of the feet, palms, and under the nails.

Stages of Melanoma

1. **Stage 0 (In Situ Melanoma):**
   - In this earliest stage, the melanoma cells are only in the outermost layer of skin and have not invaded deeper tissues. This stage is also known as "in situ," meaning "in its original place."

2. **Stage I:**
   - At this stage, the melanoma is still relatively small and may have invaded just below the outer layer of skin but not spread to nearby lymph nodes or other organs.

3. **Stage II:**
   - Melanoma has grown thicker and may have ulcerated (the skin over the tumor has broken). It still hasn't spread to lymph nodes or distant sites.

4. **Stage III:**
   - The cancer has spread to nearby lymph nodes or to the skin immediately around the original tumor.

5. **Stage IV:**
   - This is advanced melanoma, where the cancer has spread to distant lymph nodes, organs, or other parts of the skin. This stage is more challenging to treat.

Symptoms and Signs

Detecting melanoma early is crucial. The most common sign is a change in an existing mole or the development of a new, unusual-looking growth on your skin. Here's a handy guide using the ABCDE rule to identify potential melanomas:

- A for Asymmetry: One half of the mole doesn't match the other half.
- B for Border: The edges are irregular, ragged, notched, or blurred.
- C for Color: The color is not uniform and may include different shades of brown or black, sometimes with patches of pink, red, white, or blue.
- D for Diameter: The spot is larger than 6 millimeters across (about the size of a pencil eraser), although melanomas can sometimes be smaller.
- E for Evolving: The mole is changing in size, shape, or color.

Types of Melanoma

There are several types of melanoma, each with unique characteristics:

1. Superficial Spreading Melanoma:
   - This is the most common type and tends to spread across the top layer of the skin before penetrating deeper.
2. Nodular Melanoma:
   - This type is usually invasive from the start and appears as a bump. It's more aggressive and can be more challenging to treat.
3. Lentigo Maligna Melanoma:
   - Often occurring in older adults, this type develops from long-term sun exposure. It starts as a flat or slightly raised tan or brown patch that slowly darkens and enlarges.
4. Acral Lentiginous Melanoma:
   - This rare type appears on the palms, soles of the feet, or under the nails. It's more common in people with darker skin.
5. Desmoplastic Melanoma:
   - This type is rare and can be challenging to diagnose because it often appears as a scar-like lesion and lacks the typical pigmentation.

Development Over Time

The understanding and treatment of melanoma have significantly evolved over the years. Early detection through skin examinations and awareness campaigns have improved survival rates. Advancements in medical research have led to the development of targeted therapies and immunotherapies, which have proven effective in treating advanced melanoma. In the past, treatment options were limited to surgery, radiation, and conventional chemotherapy. However, the discovery of specific genetic mutations in melanoma cells has paved the way for targeted therapies that block the growth and spread of cancer by interfering with specific molecules involved in tumor growth. Immunotherapies, which stimulate the body's immune system to attack cancer cells, have also shown great promise.

Risk Factors and Prevention

Risk Factors for Melanoma
Several factors can increase the risk of developing melanoma. Some of these are controllable, while others are not. Here's a comprehensive look at the most significant risk factors:

1. Ultraviolet (UV) Light Exposure
- Sun Exposure: The primary risk factor for melanoma is exposure to ultraviolet (UV) radiation from the sun. UV rays can damage the DNA in skin cells, leading to mutations that cause melanoma.
- Tanning Beds: Artificial sources of UV radiation, such as tanning beds and sunlamps, also increase the risk. Tanning beds are particularly dangerous because they can emit UV radiation levels much higher than the sun.

2. Skin Type
- Fair Skin: People with fair skin, light hair (blonde or red), and light-colored eyes (blue or green) have less melanin, the pigment that provides some protection against UV radiation. This makes them more susceptible to skin damage from the sun.
- Freckles and Moles: Individuals with a lot of freckles or moles, especially atypical (dysplastic) moles, are at higher risk. Dysplastic moles are more likely to become melanoma than regular moles.

3. Family History and Genetics
- Family History: Having a close relative (parent, sibling, or child) with melanoma increases your risk. This suggests a genetic predisposition to melanoma.
- Genetic Mutations: Specific genetic mutations, such as those in the CDKN2A and BRAF genes, can increase the risk of developing melanoma. These mutations can be inherited or acquired over time due to UV exposure.

4. Personal History
- Previous Melanoma: If you've had melanoma before, you have a higher chance of developing it again.
- Other Skin Cancers: Having had other types of skin cancer, like basal cell carcinoma or squamous cell carcinoma, can also increase your risk.

5. Weakened Immune System
- Immunosuppression: People with weakened immune systems, such as those with HIV/AIDS or those taking immunosuppressive drugs after organ transplants, are at higher risk for melanoma and other skin cancers.

6. Age and Gender
- Age: Melanoma is more common in older adults, but it can occur at any age. It's one of the most common cancers in young adults, especially young women.
- Gender: Men have a slightly higher risk of developing melanoma than women, though women under 50 are at higher risk than men of the same age.

Prevention Strategies for Melanoma

Preventing melanoma involves reducing exposure to UV radiation, protecting your skin, and monitoring for early signs of skin changes. Here are some comprehensive strategies for prevention:

1. Sun Protection

- Use Sunscreen: Apply a broad-spectrum sunscreen with an SPF of 30 or higher to all exposed skin. Reapply every two hours, or more often if swimming or sweating.
- Wear Protective Clothing: Wear long-sleeved shirts, long pants, and wide-brimmed hats to protect your skin. Consider clothing with built-in UV protection.
- Seek Shade: Avoid direct sun exposure, especially between 10 a.m. and 4 p.m., when UV rays are strongest.
- Sunglasses: Wear sunglasses that block 100% of UVA and UVB rays to protect your eyes and the surrounding skin.

2. Avoid Tanning Beds

- Skip Tanning Beds: Avoid using tanning beds and sunlamps, as they can significantly increase your risk of melanoma.

3. Regular Skin Checks

- Self-Examinations: Perform regular self-examinations of your skin to check for new moles or changes to existing moles. Use the ABCDE rule (Asymmetry, Border, Color, Diameter, Evolving) to identify suspicious spots.
- Professional Skin Exams: See a dermatologist annually for a professional skin examination, especially if you have risk factors for melanoma.

4. Be Cautious with Medications

- Photosensitizing Medications: Some medications can make your skin more sensitive to UV radiation. Be aware of the side effects of any medications you take and take extra precautions to protect your skin if necessary.

5. Healthy Lifestyle Choices

- Healthy Diet: A diet rich in fruits, vegetables, and antioxidants can support overall skin health and potentially reduce the risk of cancer.
- Avoid Smoking: Smoking can weaken your immune system and overall health, increasing your risk of various cancers, including melanoma.

6. Education and Awareness

- Public Education: Awareness campaigns and education about the dangers of UV exposure and the importance of sun protection can help reduce melanoma rates.
- Community Programs: Community programs that provide free sunscreen, promote shade structures, and encourage protective clothing can also be effective.

Nutritional Needs for Melanoma Patients

1. Balanced Diet

A balanced diet is fundamental for everyone, but it's especially crucial for melanoma patients. A well-rounded diet helps maintain body weight, provides energy, and supplies essential nutrients needed for healing and immune function.

- Macronutrients: Ensure a proper balance of proteins, carbohydrates, and fats.
  - Proteins: Essential for repairing tissues and supporting immune function. Good sources include lean meats, fish, eggs, dairy, legumes, nuts, and seeds.
  - Carbohydrates: Provide energy, particularly important during treatment. Focus on complex carbs like whole grains, fruits, and vegetables.
  - Fats: Necessary for energy and to absorb fat-soluble vitamins. Choose healthy fats such as those from avocados, nuts, seeds, and olive oil.

2. Protein Intake

Protein is particularly important for melanoma patients due to its role in tissue repair and immune support. Treatment for melanoma, such as surgery, radiation, and chemotherapy, can increase the body's need for protein.

- High-Quality Protein Sources: Include lean meats (chicken, turkey), fish (especially fatty fish like salmon for omega-3 fatty acids), eggs, dairy products (milk, yogurt, cheese), legumes (beans, lentils), nuts, and seeds.
- Protein-Rich Snacks: Incorporate snacks like Greek yogurt, cottage cheese, hummus with veggies, or a handful of nuts.

3. Antioxidant-Rich Foods

Antioxidants help combat oxidative stress and may protect cells from damage caused by free radicals. Melanoma patients should consume a variety of antioxidant-rich foods.

- Fruits and Vegetables: Aim for a colorful plate with fruits and vegetables high in vitamins A, C, and E, and other antioxidants. Examples include berries, citrus fruits, leafy greens, bell peppers, and carrots.
- Whole Grains and Nuts: Foods like whole grains and nuts also contain beneficial antioxidants.

4. Omega-3 Fatty Acids

Omega-3 fatty acids have anti-inflammatory properties that can be beneficial for melanoma patients, as chronic inflammation can exacerbate cancer progression.

- Sources: Include fatty fish (salmon, mackerel, sardines), flaxseeds, chia seeds, walnuts, and fortified foods.

5. Vitamins and Minerals

Certain vitamins and minerals are particularly important for melanoma patients:

- Vitamin D: Important for bone health and may play a role in immune function. Sources include fatty fish, fortified dairy products, and sunlight exposure (though limited for melanoma patients due to sun sensitivity).
- Vitamin C: Supports the immune system and aids in wound healing. Found in citrus fruits, strawberries, bell peppers, and broccoli.
- Vitamin E: Acts as an antioxidant and supports skin health. Sources include nuts, seeds, and green leafy vegetables.
- Selenium: May have protective effects against cancer. Found in Brazil nuts, seafood, and whole grains.
- Zinc: Essential for immune function and wound healing. Sources include meat, shellfish, legumes, seeds, and nuts.

6. Hydration

Staying well-hydrated is crucial for all cancer patients, including those with melanoma. Proper hydration supports overall bodily functions, helps manage side effects of treatment, and maintains skin health.

- Water: Aim to drink plenty of water throughout the day.
- Hydrating Foods: Incorporate foods with high water content, such as cucumbers, melons, and soups.

7. Managing Side Effects with Nutrition

Treatment for melanoma can lead to various side effects that impact nutrition and appetite. Here are some common issues and how to address them:

- Nausea and Vomiting: Eat small, frequent meals. Try bland, easy-to-digest foods like toast, crackers, and applesauce. Ginger tea and peppermint can also help.
- Loss of Appetite: Focus on nutrient-dense foods. Smoothies, protein shakes, and meal replacement drinks can provide calories and nutrients when solid food is unappealing.
- Mouth Sores: Avoid acidic, spicy, or rough-textured foods. Opt for soft, moist foods like mashed potatoes, yogurt, and scrambled eggs.
- Fatigue: Eat small, frequent meals to keep energy levels stable. Include iron-rich foods like lean meats, spinach, and legumes to combat anemia-related fatigue.

8. Supplements

While a balanced diet is the best way to obtain nutrients, supplements can sometimes be necessary, especially if you're struggling to meet your nutritional needs through food alone. However, it's crucial to consult with a healthcare provider before starting any supplements, as some can interact with cancer treatments.

- Multivitamins: Can help fill nutritional gaps.
- Specific Supplements: Vitamin D, fish oil (omega-3s), and probiotics might be recommended based on individual needs.

9. Personalized Nutrition Plans

Each melanoma patient's nutritional needs can vary based on the stage of cancer, treatment plan, and individual health. Working with a registered dietitian who specializes in oncology can help create a personalized nutrition plan that addresses specific needs and goals.

Foods that Fight Cancer

1. Cruciferous Vegetables
Cruciferous vegetables are rich in nutrients and contain compounds that may have cancer-fighting properties.
- Broccoli: Contains sulforaphane, a compound that has been shown to reduce the size and number of cancer cells in breast, prostate, and colon cancers.
- Cauliflower: High in fiber and antioxidants, which help protect cells from damage.
- Brussels Sprouts: Contain kaempferol, an antioxidant that may reduce cancer growth.
- Cabbage: Rich in glucosinolates, which have been shown to have anti-cancer effects.
- Kale: Packed with vitamins A, C, and K, and also contains indole-3-carbinol, which may help protect against hormone-related cancers.

2. Berries
Berries are high in antioxidants and vitamins, making them powerful allies in cancer prevention.
- Blueberries: Rich in vitamins C and K, and antioxidants like anthocyanins, which may help protect cells from damage and reduce inflammation.
- Strawberries: Contain ellagic acid, which has anti-cancer properties.
- Raspberries: High in fiber and vitamin C, which support immune health and fight inflammation.
- Blackberries: Contain anthocyanins, which have been shown to reduce oxidative stress and inflammation.

3. Leafy Greens
Leafy greens are packed with vitamins, minerals, and antioxidants that support overall health and may protect against cancer.
- Spinach: Rich in vitamins A, C, and K, folate, and fiber. Contains carotenoids, which are believed to reduce cancer risk.
- Swiss Chard: High in vitamins A, C, and K, and antioxidants that help fight free radicals.
- Collard Greens: Provide a good source of fiber, vitamins, and minerals, which support overall health and may reduce cancer risk.

4. Nuts and Seeds
Nuts and seeds are rich in healthy fats, fiber, and antioxidants, which may help reduce cancer risk.
- Walnuts: Contain omega-3 fatty acids and polyphenols, which have anti-inflammatory properties and may inhibit cancer growth.
- Almonds: High in fiber, vitamin E, and healthy fats, which support immune health.

- Flaxseeds: Rich in lignans and omega-3 fatty acids, which may reduce the risk of breast cancer.
- Chia Seeds: Packed with fiber, protein, and omega-3 fatty acids, which support overall health and may have anti-cancer effects.

5. Whole Grains

Whole grains are an excellent source of fiber, vitamins, and minerals, which can help maintain a healthy weight and reduce cancer risk.

- Oats: High in fiber and beta-glucan, which supports immune health and may help lower cholesterol levels.
- Quinoa: Contains all nine essential amino acids, making it a complete protein. Also high in fiber and antioxidants.
- Brown Rice: Rich in fiber and selenium, which may reduce the risk of colon cancer.
- Barley: High in fiber and antioxidants, which support digestive health and may reduce cancer risk.

6. Legumes

Legumes are rich in fiber, protein, and antioxidants, which support overall health and may reduce cancer risk.

- Lentils: High in fiber, protein, and folate, which support immune health and may reduce cancer risk.
- Chickpeas: Packed with fiber, protein, and vitamins, which support overall health and may reduce cancer risk.
- Black Beans: Rich in fiber, protein, and antioxidants, which support digestive health and may reduce cancer risk.
- Soybeans: Contain isoflavones, which may have anti-cancer effects, particularly for hormone-related cancers.

7. Garlic and Onions

Garlic and onions contain sulfur compounds that may have cancer-fighting properties.

- Garlic: Contains allicin, which has been shown to have anti-cancer properties in studies. Regular consumption may reduce the risk of certain cancers, such as stomach and colorectal cancer.
- Onions: Rich in quercetin, an antioxidant that may have anti-inflammatory and anti-cancer effects.

8. Fish

Fatty fish are rich in omega-3 fatty acids, which have anti-inflammatory properties and may help reduce cancer risk.

- Salmon: High in omega-3 fatty acids, which support heart and brain health and may reduce inflammation.
- Mackerel: Packed with omega-3s and vitamin D, which support immune health.
- Sardines: Rich in omega-3s and calcium, which support overall health and may reduce cancer risk.

9. Citrus Fruits

Citrus fruits are rich in vitamin C and other antioxidants, which support immune health and may help protect against cancer.

- Oranges: High in vitamin C, which supports immune health and may have anti-cancer properties.
- Grapefruits: Rich in vitamin C and antioxidants, which support overall health and may reduce cancer risk.
- Lemons: Packed with vitamin C and antioxidants, which support immune health and may have anti-cancer effects.
- Limes: Rich in vitamin C and antioxidants, which support overall health and may reduce cancer risk.

10. Tomatoes

Tomatoes are rich in lycopene, an antioxidant that may help protect against certain types of cancer, particularly prostate cancer.

- Fresh Tomatoes: High in vitamins A, C, and E, and antioxidants that support overall health.
- Tomato Sauce: Cooking tomatoes increases the availability of lycopene, making tomato sauce an excellent source of this antioxidant.

11. Green Tea

Green tea is rich in catechins, antioxidants that may have anti-cancer properties.

- EGCG (Epigallocatechin Gallate): A potent catechin found in green tea that has been shown to inhibit cancer cell growth and reduce the risk of certain cancers.
- Regular Consumption: Drinking green tea regularly may support overall health and reduce cancer risk.

Foods to Avoid

1. Processed Meats
Processed meats are high in preservatives, sodium, and unhealthy fats, which can promote inflammation and potentially contribute to cancer progression.
- Examples: Bacon, sausages, hot dogs, deli meats, and ham.
- Reason to Avoid: These meats often contain nitrates and nitrites, which can form carcinogenic compounds in the body. They also tend to be high in saturated fats and sodium, which are not conducive to a healthy diet.

2. Red Meat
While red meat can be a good source of protein and iron, excessive consumption has been linked to increased cancer risk.
- Examples: Beef, pork, lamb, and veal.
- Reason to Avoid: Red meat contains heme iron, which may promote the formation of carcinogenic compounds. Cooking methods like grilling or frying can also produce carcinogens such as heterocyclic amines (HCAs) and polycyclic aromatic hydrocarbons (PAHs).

3. Sugary Foods and Beverages
High sugar intake can lead to obesity and insulin resistance, which are risk factors for many cancers, including melanoma.
- Examples: Sugary snacks (cookies, cakes, candy), sweetened beverages (soda, fruit drinks), and desserts.
- Reason to Avoid: Excess sugar contributes to weight gain and inflammation, which can compromise the immune system and promote cancer cell growth. High blood sugar levels can also feed cancer cells, which often rely on glucose for energy.

4. Refined Carbohydrates
Refined carbohydrates can spike blood sugar levels and contribute to inflammation and obesity.
- Examples: White bread, white rice, pastries, and other products made with white flour.
- Reason to Avoid: These foods have a high glycemic index, leading to rapid spikes in blood sugar and insulin levels. Over time, this can increase inflammation and the risk of developing cancer.

5. Fried and Fast Foods
Fried and fast foods are typically high in unhealthy fats, sodium, and calories, contributing to poor health outcomes.
- Examples: French fries, fried chicken, burgers, and other fast foods.
- Reason to Avoid: These foods are often cooked in unhealthy oils, leading to the formation of trans fats and other harmful compounds. They can contribute to obesity, inflammation, and increased cancer risk.

6. Alcohol

Alcohol consumption is linked to an increased risk of various cancers, including melanoma.

- Examples: Beer, wine, spirits, and cocktails.
- Reason to Avoid: Alcohol can damage DNA and interfere with the body's ability to absorb nutrients. It also promotes inflammation and can weaken the immune system, making it harder for the body to fight off cancer cells.

7. Artificial Additives and Preservatives

Artificial additives and preservatives in processed foods can have harmful effects on health.

- Examples: Artificial sweeteners, flavor enhancers (like MSG), and preservatives (like BHA and BHT).
- Reason to Avoid: These chemicals can cause allergic reactions, disrupt hormones, and may have carcinogenic effects.

8. High-Sodium Foods

High sodium intake can lead to hypertension and increased risk of heart disease, which can complicate cancer treatment and recovery.

- Examples: Processed snacks, canned soups, salty condiments, and pickled foods.
- Reason to Avoid: Excessive sodium can cause water retention and high blood pressure, putting additional strain on the cardiovascular system and overall health.

9. Foods High in Saturated and Trans Fats

Saturated and trans fats can promote inflammation and increase the risk of chronic diseases, including cancer.

- Examples: Butter, margarine, fatty cuts of meat, and packaged snacks with hydrogenated oils.
- Reason to Avoid: These fats can increase cholesterol levels, promote inflammation, and negatively impact heart health, which is crucial for overall well-being during cancer treatment.

10. Dairy Products

There is some evidence suggesting that high intake of certain dairy products may be linked to an increased risk of cancer, though the data is not conclusive.

- Examples: Whole milk, cheese, ice cream, and other high-fat dairy products.
- Reason to Limit: Some studies suggest that hormones present in dairy products might influence cancer risk. However, low-fat and fermented dairy products like yogurt can be beneficial, so moderation and balance are key.

Breakfast Recipes

1. Banana Pancakes

Ingredients:

- 1 large ripe banana
- 2 large eggs
- 1/2 teaspoon vanilla extract
- 1/2 teaspoon baking powder
- 1/4 teaspoon cinnamon
- 1/4 cup rolled oats (gluten-free if needed)
- 1 tablespoon chia seeds
- 1 tablespoon ground flaxseed
- Cooking spray (coconut oil or olive oil based)

Instructions:

1. In a blender, combine the banana, eggs, vanilla extract, baking powder, cinnamon, rolled oats, chia seeds, and ground flaxseed.
2. Blend until you have a smooth batter.
3. Heat a non-stick skillet over medium heat and lightly coat with cooking spray.
4. Pour 1/4 cup of batter onto the skillet for each pancake. Cook until bubbles form on the surface and the edges start to look set, about 2-3 minutes.
5. Flip the pancakes and cook for another 2-3 minutes until golden brown.
6. Serve warm, optionally with fresh berries and a drizzle of honey or maple syrup.

Nutrition Info (per serving):

- Calories: 180
- Protein: 8g
- Carbohydrates: 26g
- Fiber: 4g
- Sugars: 8g
- Fat: 6g
- Saturated Fat: 1g

Serves: 2

Cooking Time: 15 minutes

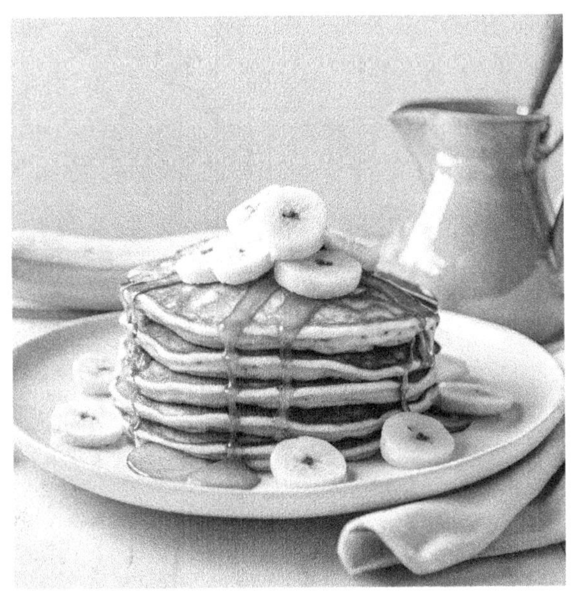

2. Oat Flour Waffles

Ingredients:

- 1 1/2 cups oat flour (can be made by blending rolled oats)
- 1 teaspoon baking powder
- 1/2 teaspoon baking soda
- 1 teaspoon cinnamon
- 1/4 teaspoon nutmeg
- 1 cup unsweetened almond milk (or any plant-based milk)
- 2 large eggs
- 2 tablespoons melted coconut oil
- 1 teaspoon vanilla extract
- 1 tablespoon ground flaxseed

Instructions:

1. Preheat your waffle iron according to the manufacturer's instructions.
2. In a large bowl, whisk together the oat flour, baking powder, baking soda, cinnamon, and nutmeg.
3. In another bowl, mix the almond milk, eggs, melted coconut oil, vanilla extract, and ground flaxseed.
4. Pour the wet ingredients into the dry ingredients and stir until just combined.
5. Lightly grease the waffle iron with cooking spray.
6. Pour the batter onto the preheated waffle iron and cook according to the manufacturer's instructions until golden brown and crispy.
7. Serve warm with fresh fruit and a dollop of Greek yogurt or a drizzle of honey.

Nutrition Info (per serving):

- Calories: 220
- Protein: 8g
- Carbohydrates: 30g
- Fiber: 5g
- Sugars: 3g
- Fat: 9g
- Saturated Fat: 4g

Serves: 4
Cooking Time: 20 minutes

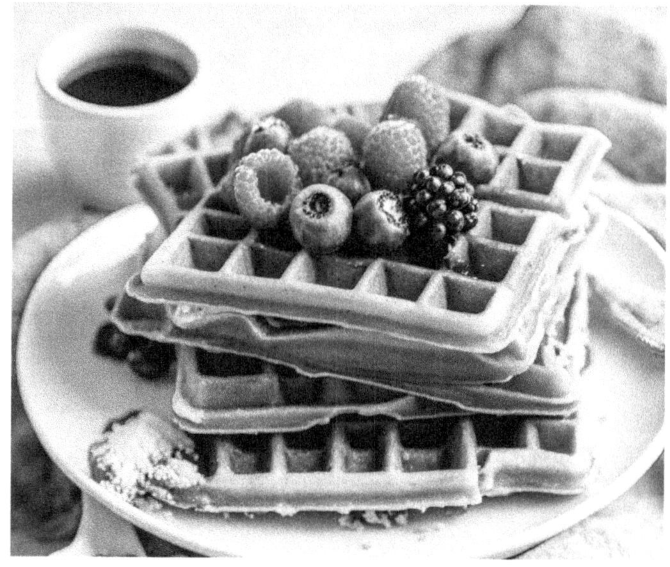

3. Cottage Cheese Pancakes

Ingredients:

- 1 cup cottage cheese (low-fat or regular)
- 3 large eggs
- 1/2 cup oat flour
- 1/4 teaspoon baking powder
- 1 teaspoon vanilla extract
- 1 tablespoon ground flaxseed
- 1/4 teaspoon cinnamon
- Cooking spray (coconut oil or olive oil based)

Instructions:

1. In a large bowl, mix together the cottage cheese, eggs, oat flour, baking powder, vanilla extract, ground flaxseed, and cinnamon until well combined.
2. Heat a non-stick skillet over medium heat and lightly coat with cooking spray.
3. Pour 1/4 cup of batter onto the skillet for each pancake. Cook until bubbles form on the surface and the edges start to look set, about 2-3 minutes.
4. Flip the pancakes and cook for another 2-3 minutes until golden brown.
5. Serve warm with a sprinkle of cinnamon and a side of fresh fruit.

Nutrition Info (per serving):

- Calories: 200
- Protein: 14g
- Carbohydrates: 20g
- Fiber: 2g
- Sugars: 5g
- Fat: 8g
- Saturated Fat: 3g

Serves: 3
Cooking Time: 15 minutes

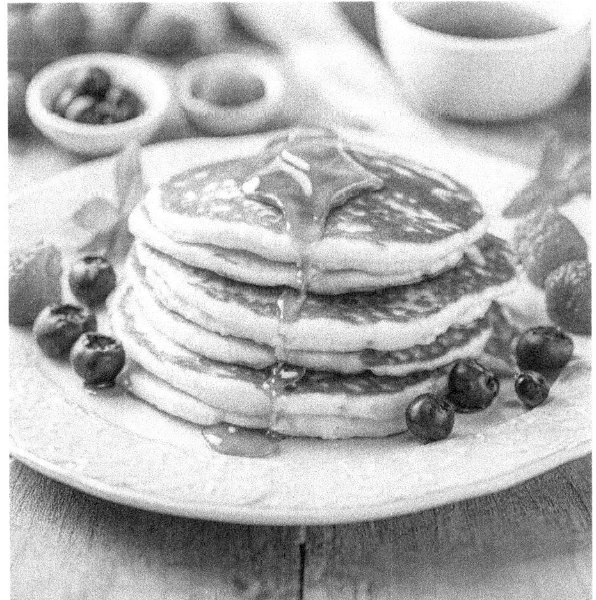

4. Breakfast Salad

Ingredients:

- 2 cups baby spinach
- 1 cup arugula
- 1/2 avocado, sliced
- 1/2 cup cherry tomatoes, halved
- 1/4 cup red bell pepper, diced
- 1/4 cup cucumber, sliced
- 2 large eggs, boiled and sliced
- 2 tablespoons pumpkin seeds
- 1 tablespoon olive oil
- 1 tablespoon lemon juice
- 1 teaspoon Dijon mustard
- 1/2 teaspoon honey
- Fresh herbs (such as parsley or basil), chopped

Instructions:

1. In a large bowl, combine the baby spinach, arugula, avocado, cherry tomatoes, red bell pepper, and cucumber.
2. Add the boiled egg slices and sprinkle with pumpkin seeds.
3. In a small bowl, whisk together the olive oil, lemon juice, Dijon mustard, and honey.
4. Drizzle the dressing over the salad and toss gently to combine.
5. Garnish with fresh herbs and serve immediately.

Nutrition Info (per serving):

- Calories: 250
- Protein: 10g
- Carbohydrates: 12g
- Fiber: 6g
- Sugars: 4g
- Fat: 20g
- Saturated Fat: 3g

Serves: 2

Cooking Time: 10 minutes

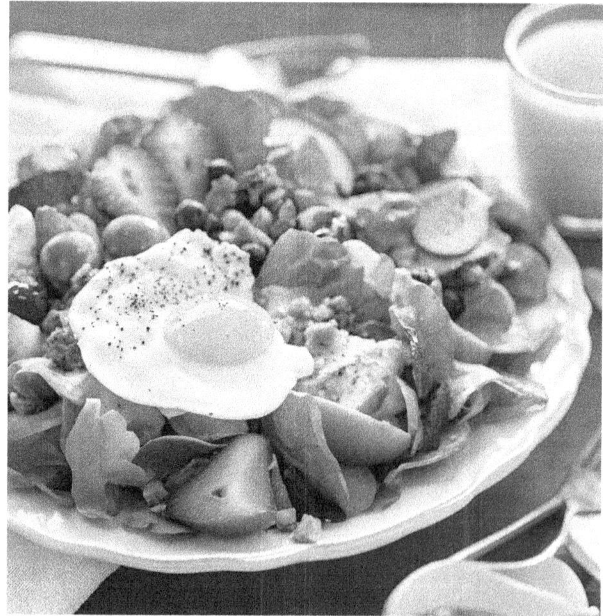

5. Almond Flour Pancakes

Ingredients:

- 1 cup almond flour
- 1/4 cup unsweetened almond milk
- 2 large eggs
- 1 tablespoon honey or maple syrup
- 1 teaspoon vanilla extract
- 1/2 teaspoon baking powder
- 1/4 teaspoon cinnamon
- Cooking spray (coconut oil or olive oil based)

Instructions:

1. In a medium bowl, whisk together the almond flour, almond milk, eggs, honey or maple syrup, vanilla extract, baking powder, and cinnamon until smooth.
2. Heat a non-stick skillet over medium heat and lightly coat with cooking spray.
3. Pour 1/4 cup of batter onto the skillet for each pancake. Cook until bubbles form on the surface and the edges start to look set, about 2-3 minutes.
4. Flip the pancakes and cook for another 2-3 minutes until golden brown.
5. Serve warm with fresh fruit and a drizzle of honey or maple syrup if desired.

Nutrition Info (per serving):

- Calories: 220
- Protein: 8g
- Carbohydrates: 12g
- Fiber: 3g
- Sugars: 5g
- Fat: 16g
- Saturated Fat: 1.5g

Serves: 4
Cooking Time: 15 minutes

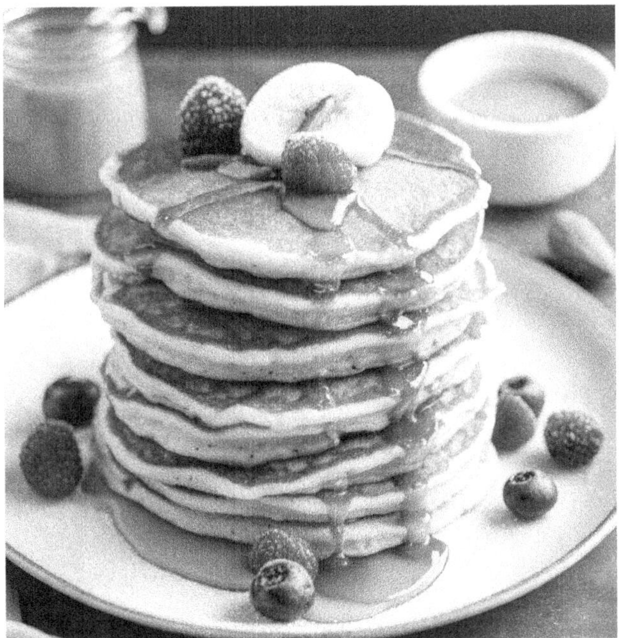

6. Buckwheat Waffles

Ingredients:

- 1 1/2 cups buckwheat flour
- 1 teaspoon baking powder
- 1/2 teaspoon baking soda
- 1 teaspoon cinnamon
- 1 cup unsweetened almond milk
- 2 large eggs
- 2 tablespoons melted coconut oil
- 1 teaspoon vanilla extract
- 1 tablespoon ground flaxseed

Instructions:

1. Preheat your waffle iron according to the manufacturer's instructions.
2. In a large bowl, whisk together the buckwheat flour, baking powder, baking soda, and cinnamon.
3. In another bowl, mix the almond milk, eggs, melted coconut oil, vanilla extract, and ground flaxseed.
4. Pour the wet ingredients into the dry ingredients and stir until just combined.
5. Lightly grease the waffle iron with cooking spray.
6. Pour the batter onto the preheated waffle iron and cook according to the manufacturer's instructions until golden brown and crispy.
7. Serve warm with fresh fruit and a drizzle of honey or maple syrup if desired.

Nutrition Info (per serving):

- Calories: 200
- Protein: 7g
- Carbohydrates: 28g
- Fiber: 4g
- Sugars: 2g
- Fat: 7g
- Saturated Fat: 3g

Serves: 4

Cooking Time: 20 minutes

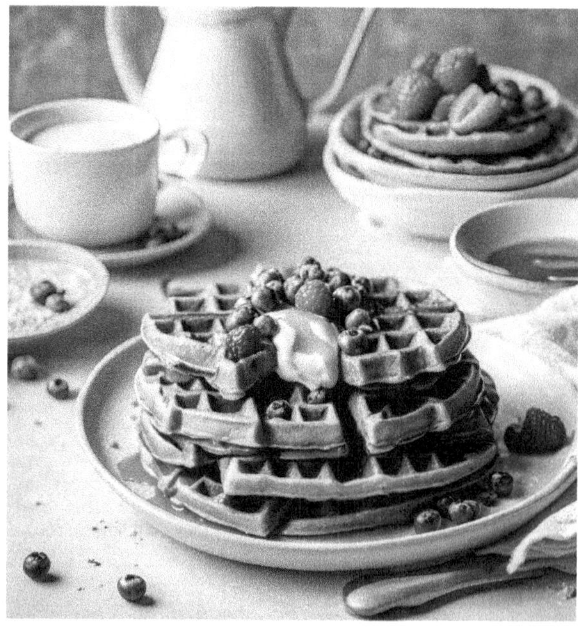

7. Sweet Corn and Zucchini Fritters

Ingredients:
- 1 cup grated zucchini (squeezed to remove excess moisture)
- 1 cup fresh or frozen corn kernels
- 1/2 cup chickpea flour
- 2 large eggs
- 1/4 cup chopped green onions
- 1/4 cup chopped fresh herbs (parsley, cilantro, or basil)
- 1/2 teaspoon cumin
- 1/4 teaspoon paprika
- Cooking spray (coconut oil or olive oil based)

Instructions:
1. In a large bowl, combine the grated zucchini, corn kernels, chickpea flour, eggs, green onions, fresh herbs, cumin, and paprika.
2. Mix well until the batter is combined.
3. Heat a non-stick skillet over medium heat and lightly coat with cooking spray.
4. Scoop 1/4 cup of batter onto the skillet for each fritter. Flatten slightly with a spatula.
5. Cook until golden brown, about 3-4 minutes per side.
6. Serve warm, optionally with a dollop of Greek yogurt or avocado slices.

Nutrition Info (per serving):
- Calories: 120
- Protein: 6g
- Carbohydrates: 14g
- Fiber: 3g
- Sugars: 3g
- Fat: 4g
- Saturated Fat: 1g

Serves: 4
Cooking Time: 20 minutes

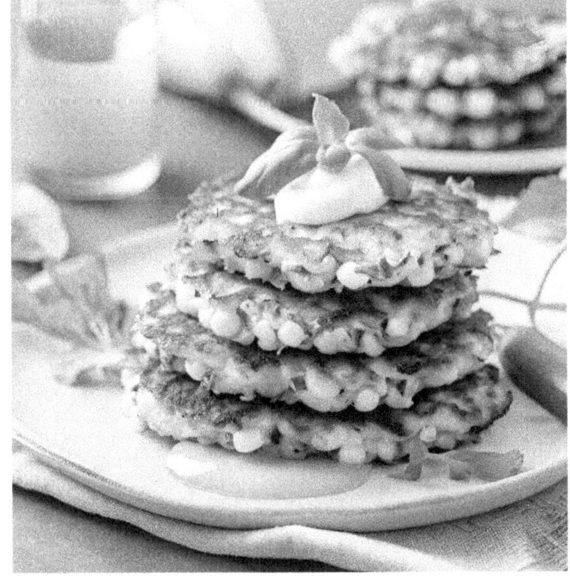

8. Millet Pudding

Ingredients:

- 1 cup millet
- 3 cups unsweetened almond milk
- 1/4 cup honey or maple syrup
- 1 teaspoon vanilla extract
- 1/2 teaspoon cinnamon
- 1/4 cup raisins or chopped dried fruit
- Fresh berries for topping (optional)

Instructions:

1. Rinse the millet under cold water.
2. In a medium saucepan, combine the millet and almond milk. Bring to a boil, then reduce the heat to low and simmer for 20-25 minutes, stirring occasionally, until the millet is tender and the mixture is thickened.
3. Stir in the honey or maple syrup, vanilla extract, cinnamon, and raisins or dried fruit.
4. Cook for an additional 5 minutes, stirring frequently.
5. Serve warm or chilled, topped with fresh berries if desired.

Nutrition Info (per serving):

- Calories: 210
- Protein: 5g
- Carbohydrates: 40g
- Fiber: 3g
- Sugars: 15g
- Fat: 3g
- Saturated Fat: 0.5g

Serves: 4

Cooking Time: 30 minutes

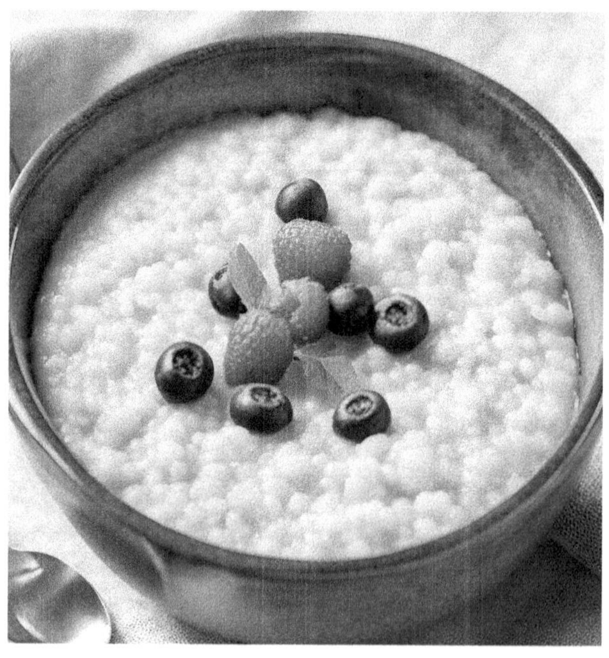

9. Pumpkin Seed Granola

Ingredients:

- 2 cups rolled oats (gluten-free if needed)
- 1 cup raw pumpkin seeds
- 1/2 cup unsweetened shredded coconut
- 1/4 cup chia seeds
- 1/4 cup ground flaxseed
- 1/4 cup honey or maple syrup
- 1/4 cup melted coconut oil
- 1 teaspoon vanilla extract
- 1 teaspoon cinnamon

Instructions:

1. Preheat the oven to 300°F (150°C) and line a baking sheet with parchment paper.
2. In a large bowl, mix together the rolled oats, pumpkin seeds, shredded coconut, chia seeds, and ground flaxseed.
3. In a small bowl, whisk together the honey or maple syrup, melted coconut oil, vanilla extract, and cinnamon.
4. Pour the wet mixture over the dry ingredients and stir until well combined.
5. Spread the mixture evenly on the prepared baking sheet.
6. Bake for 25-30 minutes, stirring halfway through, until golden brown.
7. Allow the granola to cool completely before storing in an airtight container.

Nutrition Info (per serving):

- Calories: 220
- Protein: 6g
- Carbohydrates: 24g
- Fiber: 5g
- Sugars: 8g
- Fat: 12g
- Saturated Fat: 5g

Serves: 8

Cooking Time: 35 minutes

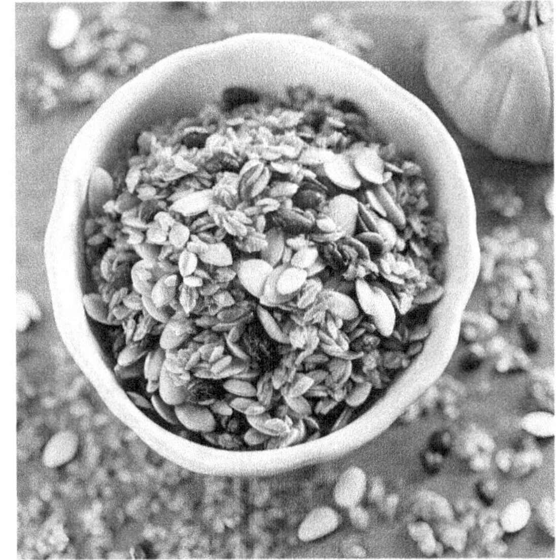

10. Soy Yogurt with Granola

Ingredients:

- 1 cup unsweetened soy yogurt
- 1/4 cup homemade pumpkin seed granola (see recipe above)
- 1/2 cup mixed berries (strawberries, blueberries, raspberries)
- 1 tablespoon chia seeds
- 1 teaspoon honey or maple syrup (optional)

Instructions:

1. In a serving bowl, spoon the soy yogurt.
2. Top with the homemade pumpkin seed granola.
3. Add the mixed berries on top.
4. Sprinkle with chia seeds.
5. Drizzle with honey or maple syrup if desired.

Nutrition Info (per serving):

- Calories: 250
- Protein: 10g
- Carbohydrates: 30g
- Fiber: 6g
- Sugars: 12g
- Fat: 10g
- Saturated Fat: 2g

Serves: 1

Cooking Time: 5 minutes

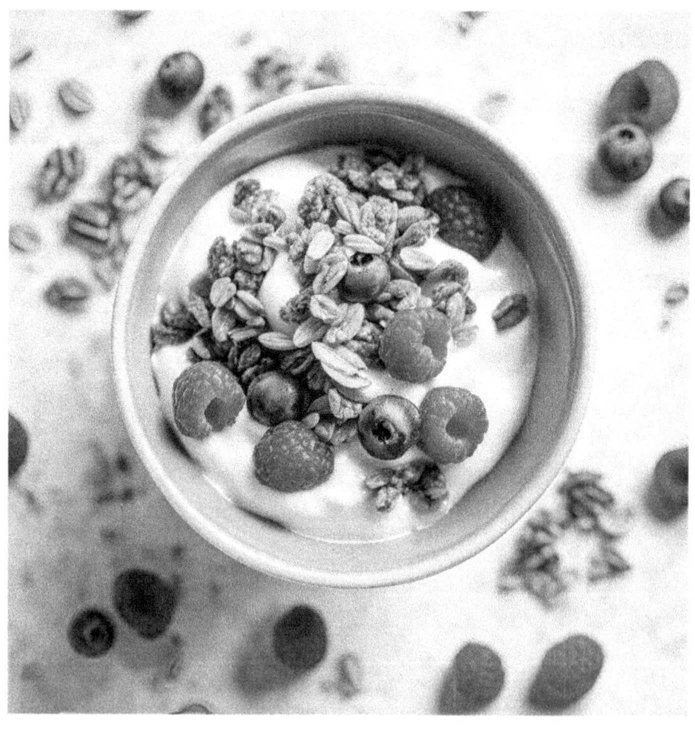

11. Congee

Ingredients:

- 1 cup jasmine rice
- 8 cups water or low-sodium vegetable broth
- 1-inch piece of ginger, sliced
- 2 cloves garlic, minced
- 1 cup chopped mushrooms
- 1/2 cup grated carrots
- 2 green onions, chopped
- 1 tablespoon soy sauce (low-sodium)
- Fresh cilantro for garnish

Instructions:

1. Rinse the rice under cold water until the water runs clear.
2. In a large pot, bring the water or broth to a boil.
3. Add the rice, ginger, and garlic. Reduce heat to low and simmer, stirring occasionally, until the rice breaks down and the mixture becomes creamy, about 1-1.5 hours.
4. Add the mushrooms and carrots in the last 15 minutes of cooking.
5. Stir in the soy sauce and green onions before serving.
6. Garnish with fresh cilantro.

Nutrition Info (per serving):

- Calories: 150
- Protein: 4g
- Carbohydrates: 30g
- Fiber: 2g
- Sugars: 2g
- Fat: 2g
- Saturated Fat: 0g

Serves: 6

Cooking Time: 1.5 hours

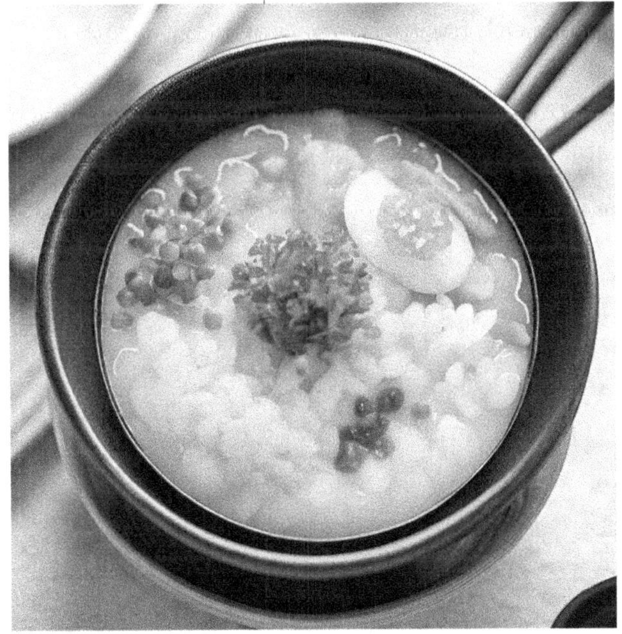

12. Masala Dosa

Ingredients:

- 1 cup dosa batter (store-bought or homemade)
- 2 medium potatoes, boiled and mashed
- 1/2 cup chopped onions
- 1/2 cup chopped tomatoes
- 1/2 teaspoon turmeric powder
- 1 teaspoon mustard seeds
- 1 teaspoon cumin seeds
- 2 tablespoons olive oil
- 1/2 teaspoon curry powder
- Fresh cilantro for garnish

Instructions:

1. Heat 1 tablespoon of olive oil in a pan over medium heat. Add mustard seeds and cumin seeds. Let them splutter.
2. Add chopped onions and sauté until golden brown.
3. Add tomatoes, turmeric powder, and curry powder. Cook until the tomatoes are soft.
4. Add the mashed potatoes and mix well. Cook for another 5 minutes. Set aside.
5. Heat a non-stick skillet over medium-high heat. Lightly coat with the remaining olive oil.
6. Pour a ladleful of dosa batter onto the skillet and spread it thinly.
7. Cook until the edges start to lift and the bottom is golden brown.
8. Place a portion of the potato filling in the center of the dosa and fold over.
9. Serve hot with fresh cilantro garnish.

Nutrition Info (per serving):

- Calories: 200
- Protein: 5g
- Carbohydrates: 32g
- Fiber: 4g
- Sugars: 4g
- Fat: 7g
- Saturated Fat: 1g

Serves: 4

Cooking Time: 30 minutes

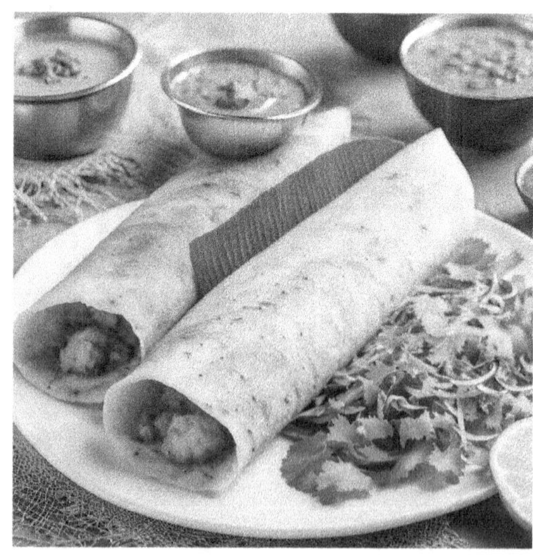

13. Japanese Breakfast Bowl

Ingredients:

- 1 cup cooked brown rice
- 1/2 avocado, sliced
- 1 cup steamed spinach
- 1 sheet nori (seaweed), cut into strips
- 1 tablespoon sesame seeds
- 1 teaspoon sesame oil
- 1 tablespoon low-sodium soy sauce
- Pickled ginger for garnish

Instructions:

1. In a bowl, arrange the cooked brown rice.
2. Top with sliced avocado, steamed spinach, and nori strips.
3. Sprinkle sesame seeds over the top.
4. Drizzle with sesame oil and soy sauce.
5. Garnish with pickled ginger.

Nutrition Info (per serving):

- Calories: 300
- Protein: 7g
- Carbohydrates: 40g
- Fiber: 7g
- Sugars: 2g
- Fat: 14g
- Saturated Fat: 2g

Serves: 1
Cooking Time: 15 minutes

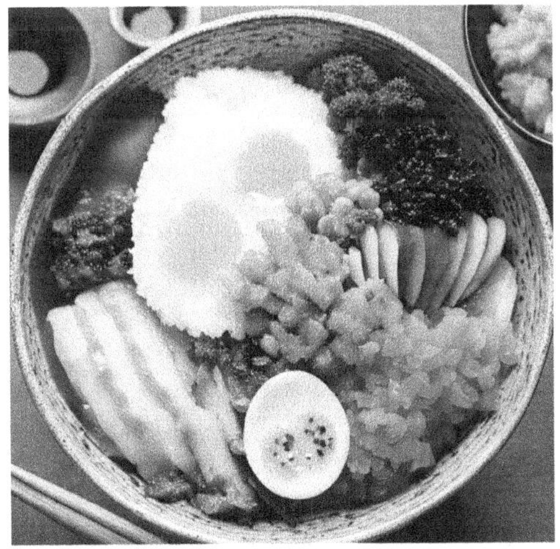

14. Chia and Coconut Rice Pudding

Ingredients:

- 1/2 cup cooked brown rice
- 1 cup unsweetened coconut milk
- 2 tablespoons chia seeds
- 1 tablespoon honey or maple syrup
- 1 teaspoon vanilla extract
- Fresh berries for topping

Instructions:

1. In a saucepan, combine the cooked brown rice, coconut milk, chia seeds, honey or maple syrup, and vanilla extract.
2. Cook over medium heat, stirring frequently, until the mixture thickens, about 10-15 minutes.
3. Serve warm or chilled, topped with fresh berries.

Nutrition Info (per serving):

- Calories: 250
- Protein: 4g
- Carbohydrates: 32g
- Fiber: 5g
- Sugars: 10g
- Fat: 12g
- Saturated Fat: 10g

Serves: 2

Cooking Time: 15 minutes

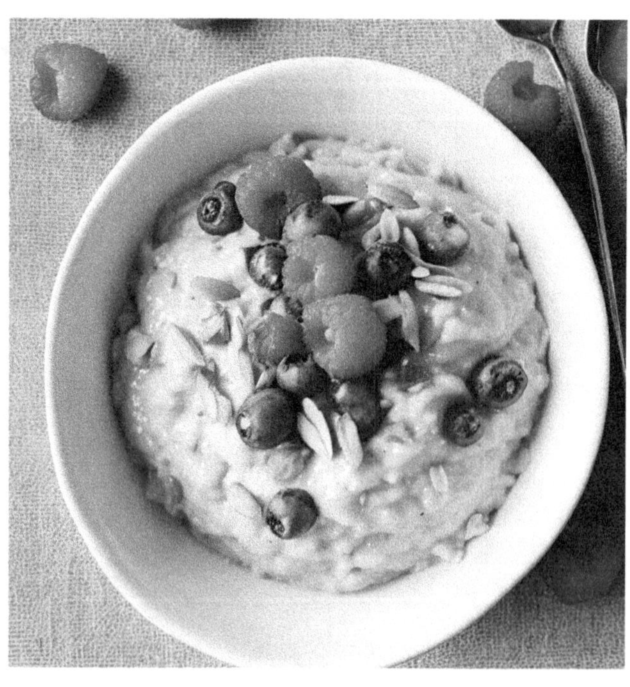

15. Baked Pears with Walnuts

Ingredients:

- 2 ripe pears, halved and cored
- 1/4 cup chopped walnuts
- 1 tablespoon honey or maple syrup
- 1/2 teaspoon cinnamon
- 1/4 teaspoon nutmeg

Instructions:

1. Preheat the oven to 350°F (175°C).
2. Place the pear halves in a baking dish, cut side up.
3. Sprinkle chopped walnuts over the pears.
4. Drizzle with honey or maple syrup and sprinkle with cinnamon and nutmeg.
5. Bake for 20-25 minutes, until the pears are tender.
6. Serve warm.

Nutrition Info (per serving):

- Calories: 180
- Protein: 2g
- Carbohydrates: 24g
- Fiber: 5g
- Sugars: 15g
- Fat: 9g
- Saturated Fat: 1g

Serves: 4
Cooking Time: 30 minutes

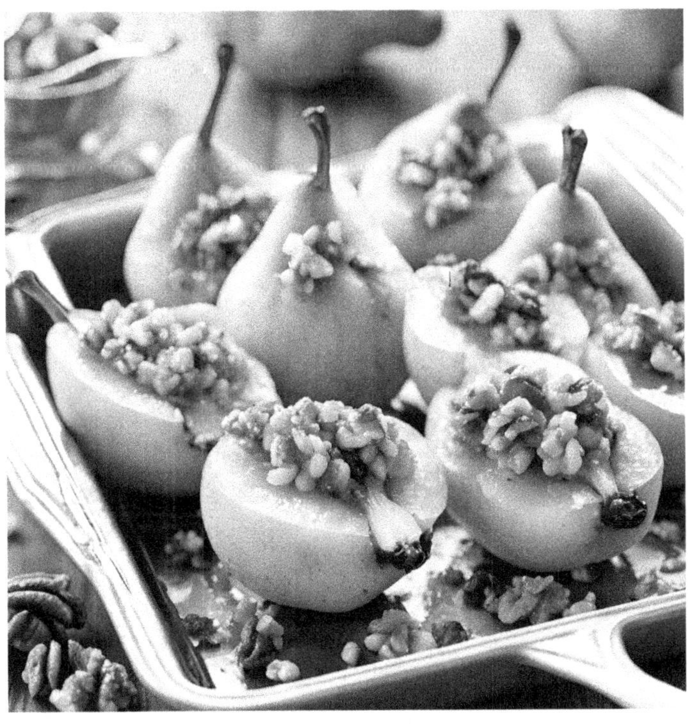

16. Cucumber and Hummus Plate

Ingredients:

- 1 large cucumber, sliced
- 1 cup hummus (store-bought or homemade)
- 1/4 cup cherry tomatoes, halved
- 1/4 cup sliced red bell pepper
- 1 tablespoon olive oil
- 1 teaspoon paprika
- Fresh parsley for garnish

Instructions:

1. Arrange the cucumber slices, cherry tomatoes, and red bell pepper on a serving plate.
2. Place the hummus in the center of the plate.
3. Drizzle the olive oil over the hummus and sprinkle with paprika.
4. Garnish with fresh parsley.

Nutrition Info (per serving):

- Calories: 180
- Protein: 6g
- Carbohydrates: 18g
- Fiber: 6g
- Sugars: 5g
- Fat: 10g
- Saturated Fat: 1g

Serves: 2
Cooking Time: 10 minutes

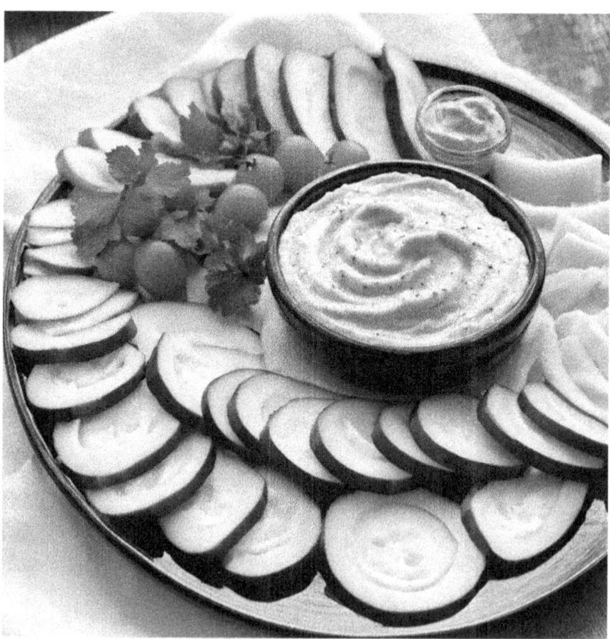

17. Blueberry Spinach Smoothie

Ingredients:

- 1 cup fresh spinach
- 1 cup frozen blueberries
- 1 banana
- 1 cup unsweetened almond milk
- 1 tablespoon chia seeds
- 1 teaspoon honey or maple syrup (optional)

Instructions:

1. Place all ingredients in a blender.
2. Blend until smooth and creamy.
3. Pour into a glass and serve immediately.

Nutrition Info (per serving):

Calories: 180   Protein: 3g   Carbohydrates: 35g   Fiber: 7g   Sugars: 18g

- Fat: 4g
- Saturated Fat: 0g

Serves: 1
Cooking Time: 5 minutes

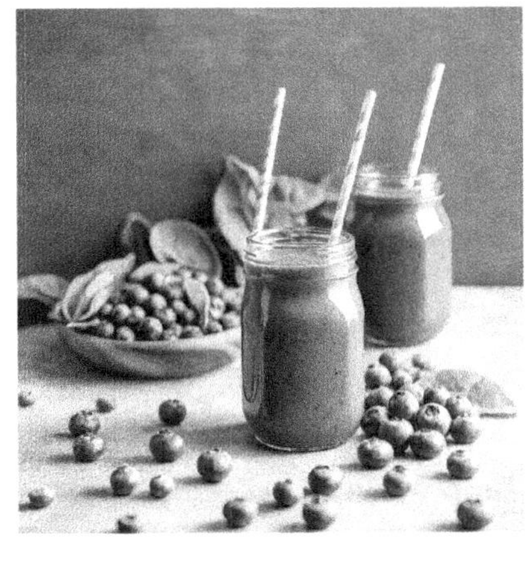

18. Avocado Green Smoothie

Ingredients:

- 1/2 avocado
- 1 cup fresh spinach
- 1/2 cucumber, peeled and chopped
- 1 green apple, cored and chopped
- 1 cup unsweetened coconut water
- 1 tablespoon ground flaxseed
- Juice of 1/2 lime

Instructions:

1. Place all ingredients in a blender.
2. Blend until smooth and creamy.
3. Pour into a glass and serve immediately.

Nutrition Info (per serving):

- Calories: 220
- Protein: 3g
- Carbohydrates: 30g
- Fiber: 10g
- Sugars: 14g
- Fat: 12g
- Saturated Fat: 2g

Serves: 1
Cooking Time: 5 minutes

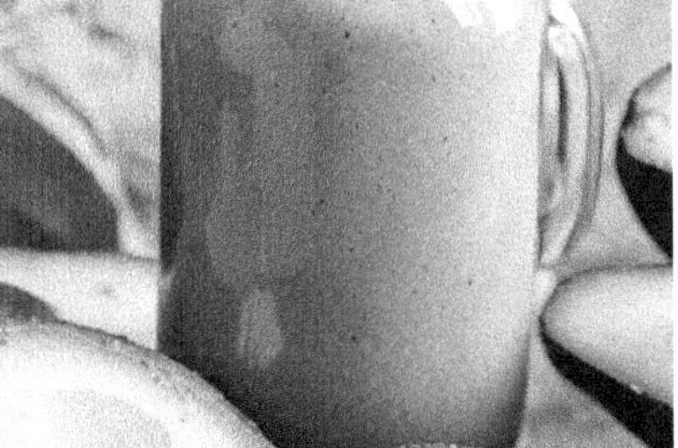

19. Buckwheat Porridge

Ingredients:

- 1 cup buckwheat groats
- 3 cups water
- 1/2 cup unsweetened almond milk
- 1 tablespoon honey or maple syrup
- 1 teaspoon vanilla extract
- 1/2 teaspoon cinnamon
- Fresh berries for topping (optional)

Instructions:

1. Rinse the buckwheat groats under cold water.
2. In a medium saucepan, bring the water to a boil.
3. Add the buckwheat groats, reduce heat, and simmer for 15-20 minutes, until the water is absorbed and the groats are tender.
4. Stir in the almond milk, honey or maple syrup, vanilla extract, and cinnamon.
5. Cook for an additional 5 minutes, stirring frequently.
6. Serve warm, topped with fresh berries if desired.

Nutrition Info (per serving):

- Calories: 240
- Protein: 6g
- Carbohydrates: 50g
- Fiber: 8g
- Sugars: 10g
- Fat: 3g
- Saturated Fat: 0g

Serves: 4
Cooking Time: 25 minutes

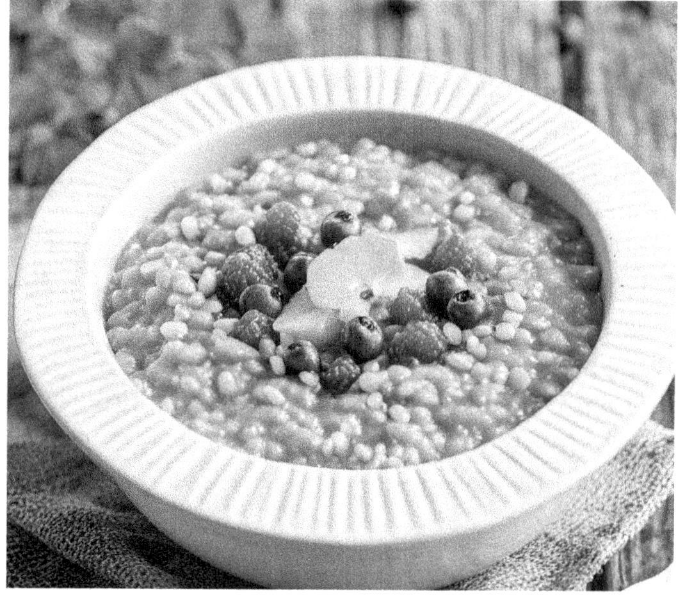

20. Quinoa Porridge

Ingredients:

- 1 cup quinoa
- 2 cups water
- 1 cup unsweetened almond milk
- 1 tablespoon honey or maple syrup
- 1 teaspoon vanilla extract
- 1/2 teaspoon cinnamon
- 1/4 cup chopped nuts (almonds, walnuts, or pecans)
- Fresh fruit for topping (optional)

Instructions:

1. Rinse the quinoa under cold water.
2. In a medium saucepan, bring the water to a boil.
3. Add the quinoa, reduce heat, and simmer for 15 minutes, until the water is absorbed and the quinoa is tender.
4. Stir in the almond milk, honey or maple syrup, vanilla extract, and cinnamon.
5. Cook for an additional 5 minutes, stirring frequently.
6. Serve warm, topped with chopped nuts and fresh fruit if desired.

Nutrition Info (per serving):

- Calories: 250
- Protein: 8g
- Carbohydrates: 38g
- Fiber: 5g
- Sugars: 10g
- Fat: 8g
- Saturated Fat: 1g

Serves: 4
Cooking Time: 20 minutes

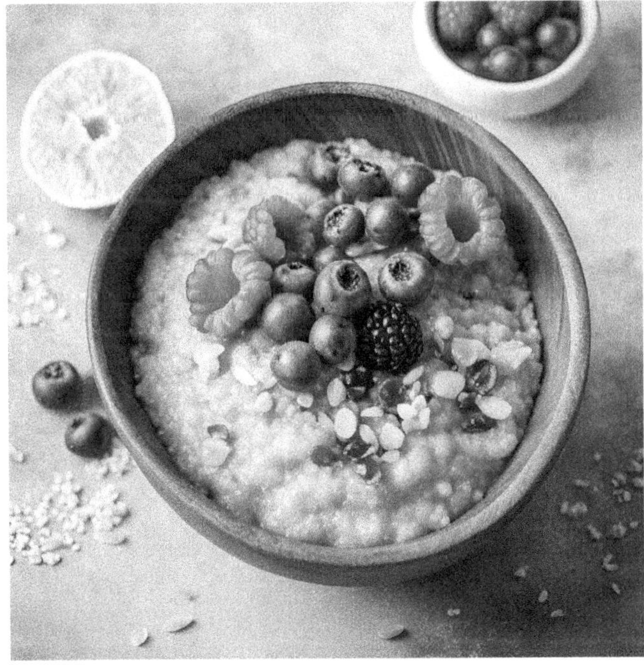

21. Tomato Basil Bruschetta

Ingredients:

- 4 ripe tomatoes, diced
- 1/4 cup fresh basil, chopped
- 2 cloves garlic, minced
- 1 tablespoon balsamic vinegar
- 1 tablespoon olive oil
- 1 whole-grain baguette, sliced
- 1 teaspoon dried oregano

Instructions:

1. Preheat the oven to 400°F (200°C).
2. In a medium bowl, combine the diced tomatoes, fresh basil, garlic, balsamic vinegar, olive oil, and dried oregano.
3. Arrange the baguette slices on a baking sheet and toast in the oven for 5-7 minutes, until golden brown.
4. Spoon the tomato mixture onto the toasted baguette slices.
5. Serve immediately.

Nutrition Info (per serving):

- Calories: 150
- Protein: 4g
- Carbohydrates: 20g
- Fiber: 3g
- Sugars: 4g
- Fat: 6g
- Saturated Fat: 1g

Serves: 6

Cooking Time: 15 minutes

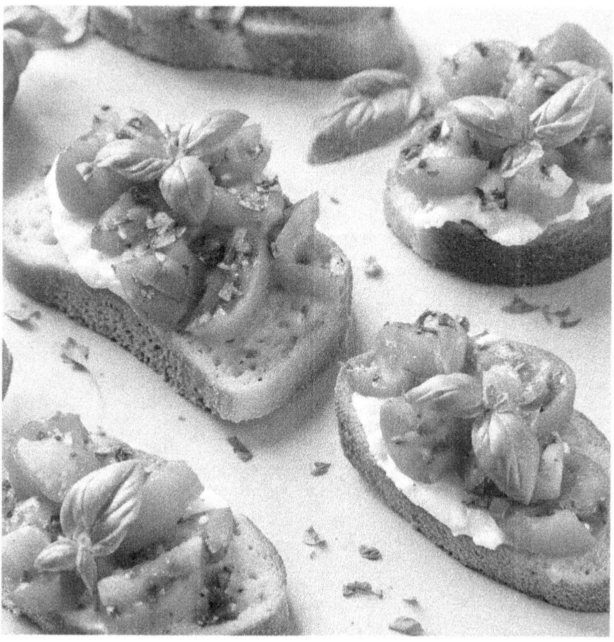

22. Ricotta & Fig Toast

Ingredients:

- 4 slices whole-grain bread
- 1 cup ricotta cheese (low-fat or regular)
- 4 fresh figs, sliced
- 1 tablespoon honey
- 1 teaspoon chopped fresh rosemary

Instructions:

1. Toast the whole-grain bread slices until golden brown.
2. Spread 1/4 cup of ricotta cheese on each slice of toast.
3. Arrange the fig slices on top of the ricotta cheese.
4. Drizzle each toast with honey and sprinkle with chopped fresh rosemary.
5. Serve immediately.

Nutrition Info (per serving):

- Calories: 200
- Protein: 9g
- Carbohydrates: 28g
- Fiber: 4g
- Sugars: 12g
- Fat: 6g
- Saturated Fat: 3g

Serves: 4
Cooking Time: 10 minutes

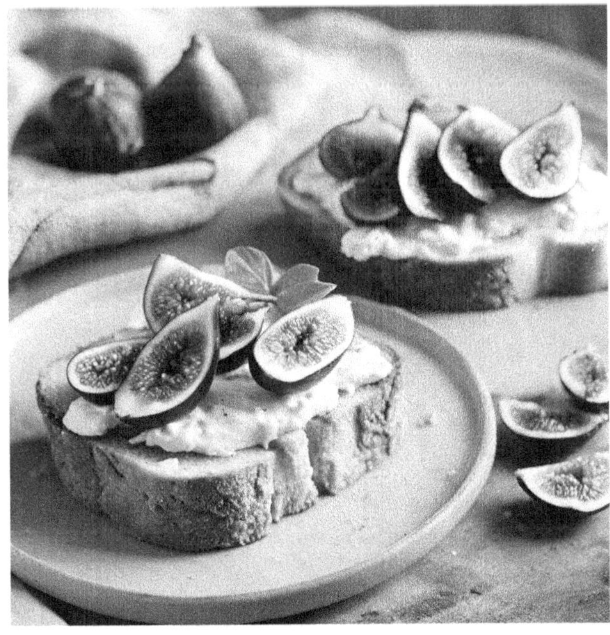

23. Mushroom & Spinach Toast

Ingredients:

- 4 slices whole-grain bread
- 1 cup sliced mushrooms (any variety)
- 2 cups fresh spinach
- 2 cloves garlic, minced
- 2 tablespoons olive oil
- 1/4 teaspoon thyme
- 1 tablespoon lemon juice

Instructions:

1. Toast the whole-grain bread slices until golden brown.
2. In a large skillet, heat the olive oil over medium heat.
3. Add the garlic and cook for 1 minute until fragrant.
4. Add the mushrooms and thyme, cooking until the mushrooms are tender, about 5 minutes.
5. Add the fresh spinach and cook until wilted, about 2-3 minutes.
6. Stir in the lemon juice.
7. Spoon the mushroom and spinach mixture over the toasted bread slices.
8. Serve immediately.

Nutrition Info (per serving):

- Calories: 180
- Protein: 6g
- Carbohydrates: 22g
- Fiber: 4g
- Sugars: 3g
- Fat: 9g
- Saturated Fat: 1.5g

Serves: 4
Cooking Time: 15 minutes

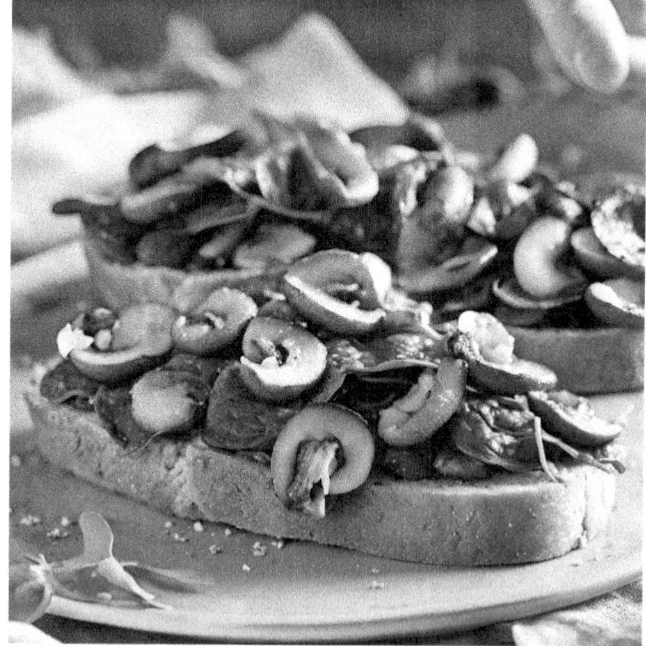

24. Frittata with Asparagus

Ingredients:

- 8 large eggs
- 1/4 cup unsweetened almond milk
- 1 cup chopped asparagus
- 1/2 cup chopped red bell pepper
- 1/2 cup chopped onions
- 1/4 cup chopped fresh parsley
- 2 tablespoons olive oil
- 1/2 teaspoon paprika

Instructions:

1. Preheat the oven to 375°F (190°C).
2. In a large bowl, whisk together the eggs and almond milk.
3. In a large oven-safe skillet, heat the olive oil over medium heat.
4. Add the onions and cook until translucent, about 3 minutes.
5. Add the asparagus and red bell pepper, cooking until tender, about 5-7 minutes.
6. Pour the egg mixture over the vegetables and stir gently to combine.
7. Cook on the stovetop for 2-3 minutes until the edges start to set.
8. Transfer the skillet to the preheated oven and bake for 15-20 minutes, until the frittata is fully set and golden brown.
9. Sprinkle with chopped fresh parsley and paprika before serving.

Nutrition Info (per serving):

- Calories: 180
- Protein: 11g
- Carbohydrates: 6g
- Fiber: 2g
- Sugars: 3g
- Fat: 13g
- Saturated Fat: 3g

Serves: 6

Cooking Time: 30 minutes

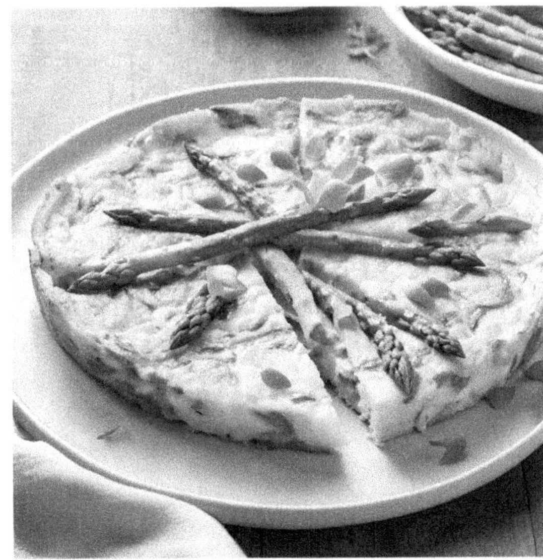

25. Sweet Potato Bowl

Ingredients:

- 2 large sweet potatoes, peeled and cubed
- 1 cup cooked quinoa
- 1 avocado, sliced
- 1 cup black beans, rinsed and drained
- 1/2 cup cherry tomatoes, halved
- 2 tablespoons olive oil
- 1 teaspoon cumin
- 1/4 teaspoon paprika
- Juice of 1 lime
- Fresh cilantro for garnish

Instructions:

1. Preheat the oven to 400°F (200°C).
2. Toss the cubed sweet potatoes with 1 tablespoon of olive oil, cumin, and paprika. Spread on a baking sheet.
3. Roast in the preheated oven for 25-30 minutes, until tender and golden brown.
4. In a bowl, combine the cooked quinoa, black beans, cherry tomatoes, and roasted sweet potatoes.
5. Drizzle with the remaining olive oil and lime juice, and toss gently to combine.
6. Top with sliced avocado and garnish with fresh cilantro.
7. Serve immediately.

Nutrition Info (per serving):

- Calories: 350
- Protein: 8g
- Carbohydrates: 45g
- Fiber: 10g
- Sugars: 6g
- Fat: 18g
- Saturated Fat: 2.5g

Serves: 4
Cooking Time: 35 minutes

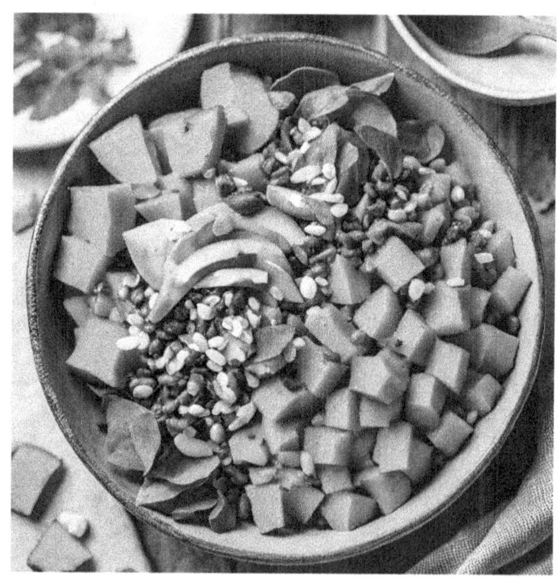

Vegetables

1. Kale and Quinoa Salad

Ingredients:

- 1 cup quinoa
- 2 cups water
- 4 cups chopped kale (stems removed)
- 1/2 cup diced red bell pepper
- 1/2 cup shredded carrots
- 1/4 cup chopped red onion
- 1/4 cup sunflower seeds
- 1/4 cup dried cranberries (unsweetened)
- 1/4 cup olive oil
- 2 tablespoons lemon juice
- 1 tablespoon Dijon mustard
- 1 tablespoon honey or maple syrup
- 1 teaspoon cumin

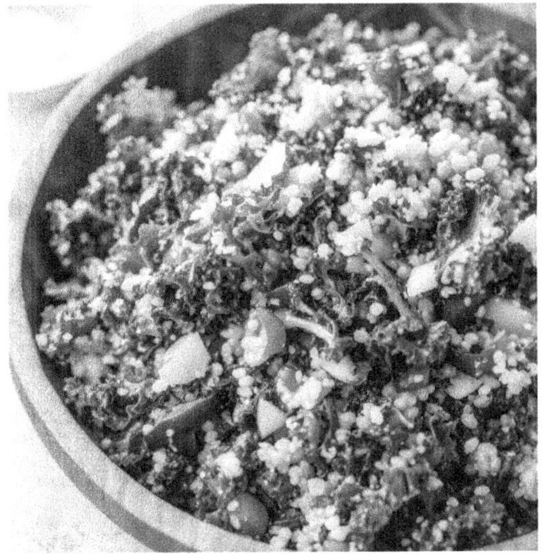

Instructions:

1. Rinse the quinoa under cold water. In a medium saucepan, bring the water to a boil.
2. Add the quinoa, reduce heat, and simmer for 15 minutes, until the water is absorbed and the quinoa is tender. Let cool.
3. In a large bowl, combine the kale, red bell pepper, shredded carrots, and red onion.
4. Add the cooked quinoa, sunflower seeds, and dried cranberries to the bowl.
5. In a small bowl, whisk together the olive oil, lemon juice, Dijon mustard, honey or maple syrup, and cumin.
6. Pour the dressing over the salad and toss well to combine.
7. Serve immediately or refrigerate for later.

Nutrition Info (per serving):

- Calories: 250
- Protein: 6g
- Carbohydrates: 32g
- Fiber: 5g
- Sugars: 8g
- Fat: 12g
- Saturated Fat: 1.5g

Serves: 4

Cooking Time: 25 minutes

2. Broccoli Salad

Ingredients:

- 4 cups broccoli florets
- 1/2 cup shredded carrots
- 1/4 cup chopped red onion
- 1/4 cup sunflower seeds
- 1/4 cup raisins
- 1/2 cup Greek yogurt
- 2 tablespoons apple cider vinegar
- 1 tablespoon honey or maple syrup
- 1 teaspoon Dijon mustard

Instructions:

1. Steam the broccoli florets for 3-4 minutes until just tender. Let cool.
2. In a large bowl, combine the cooled broccoli, shredded carrots, chopped red onion, sunflower seeds, and raisins.
3. In a small bowl, whisk together the Greek yogurt, apple cider vinegar, honey or maple syrup, and Dijon mustard.
4. Pour the dressing over the salad and toss well to combine.
5. Serve immediately or refrigerate for later.

Nutrition Info (per serving):

- Calories: 150
- Protein: 5g
- Carbohydrates: 22g
- Fiber: 5g
- Sugars: 12g
- Fat: 5g
- Saturated Fat: 1g

Serves: 4
Cooking Time: 10 minutes

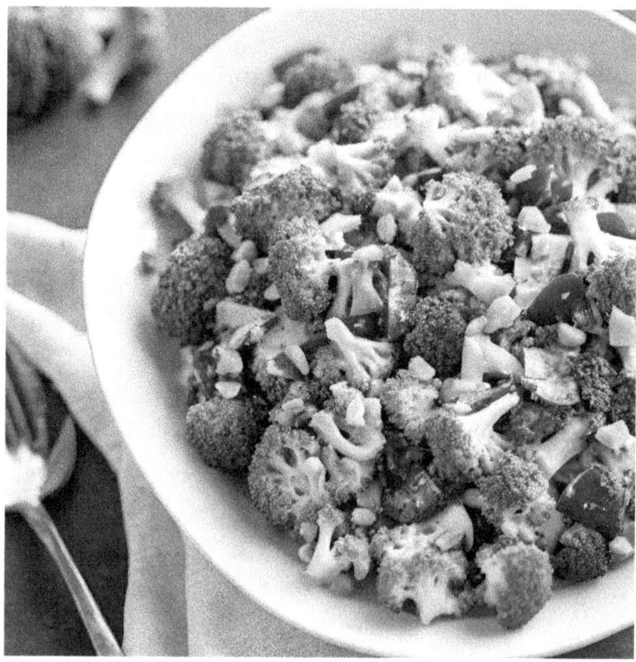

3. Carrot and Apple Slaw

Ingredients:

- 2 cups shredded carrots
- 2 apples, julienned
- 1/4 cup chopped fresh parsley
- 1/4 cup sunflower seeds
- 1/4 cup raisins
- 2 tablespoons olive oil
- 2 tablespoons lemon juice
- 1 tablespoon honey or maple syrup
- 1/2 teaspoon ground cumin

Instructions:

1. In a large bowl, combine the shredded carrots, julienned apples, chopped parsley, sunflower seeds, and raisins.
2. In a small bowl, whisk together the olive oil, lemon juice, honey or maple syrup, and ground cumin.
3. Pour the dressing over the slaw and toss well to combine.
4. Serve immediately or refrigerate for later.

Nutrition Info (per serving):

- Calories: 140
- Protein: 2g
- Carbohydrates: 21g
- Fiber: 4g
- Sugars: 14g
- Fat: 6g
- Saturated Fat: 1g

Serves: 4
Cooking Time: 10 minutes

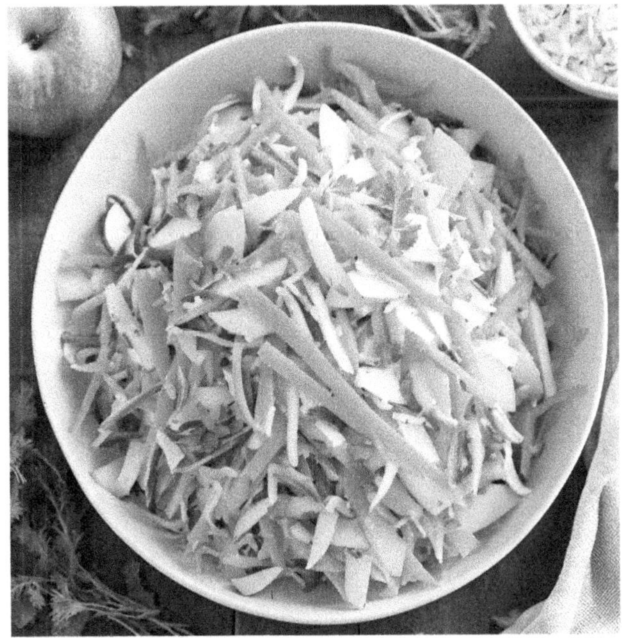

4. Asian Cabbage Salad

Ingredients:

- 4 cups shredded green cabbage
- 1 cup shredded red cabbage
- 1 cup shredded carrots
- 1/4 cup chopped green onions
- 1/4 cup chopped fresh cilantro
- 1/4 cup sliced almonds
- 1 tablespoon sesame seeds
- 1/4 cup olive oil
- 2 tablespoons rice vinegar
- 1 tablespoon soy sauce (low-sodium)
- 1 tablespoon honey or maple syrup
- 1 teaspoon sesame oil

Instructions:

1. In a large bowl, combine the shredded green cabbage, red cabbage, shredded carrots, chopped green onions, and chopped cilantro.
2. Add the sliced almonds and sesame seeds to the bowl.
3. In a small bowl, whisk together the olive oil, rice vinegar, soy sauce, honey or maple syrup, and sesame oil.
4. Pour the dressing over the salad and toss well to combine.
5. Serve immediately or refrigerate for later.

Nutrition Info (per serving):

- Calories: 180
- Protein: 4g
- Carbohydrates: 15g
- Fiber: 5g
- Sugars: 8g
- Fat: 12g
- Saturated Fat: 1.5g

Serves: 4

Cooking Time: 10 minutes

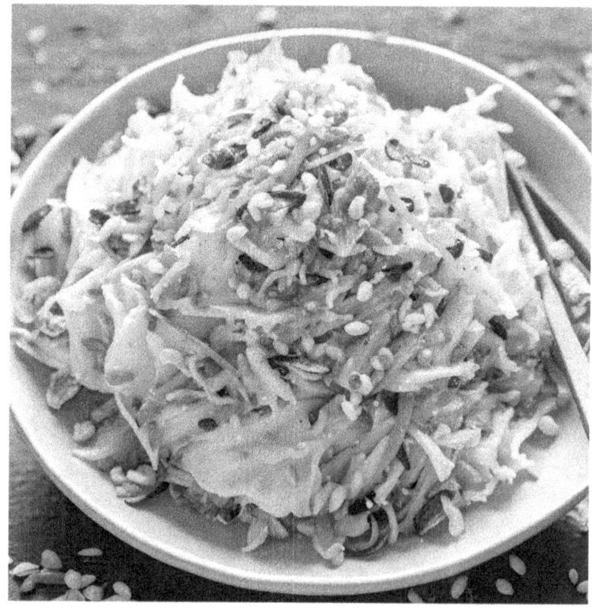

5. Tomato Basil Soup

Ingredients:

- 1 tablespoon olive oil
- 1 large onion, chopped
- 2 cloves garlic, minced
- 4 cups chopped fresh tomatoes (or 2 cans diced tomatoes, no salt added)
- 2 cups low-sodium vegetable broth
- 1/2 cup chopped fresh basil
- 1 teaspoon dried oregano
- 1/2 teaspoon ground black pepper
- 1 tablespoon balsamic vinegar

Instructions:

1. Heat the olive oil in a large pot over medium heat.
2. Add the chopped onion and cook until translucent, about 5 minutes.
3. Add the garlic and cook for another 1 minute.
4. Stir in the chopped tomatoes, vegetable broth, basil, oregano, and black pepper.
5. Bring to a boil, then reduce heat and simmer for 20 minutes.
6. Use an immersion blender to puree the soup until smooth, or carefully transfer to a blender in batches and blend until smooth.
7. Stir in the balsamic vinegar and cook for another 5 minutes.
8. Serve hot.

Nutrition Info (per serving):

- Calories: 120
- Protein: 3g
- Carbohydrates: 18g
- Fiber: 4g
- Sugars: 12g
- Fat: 4g
- Saturated Fat: 0.5g

Serves: 4

Cooking Time: 30 minutes

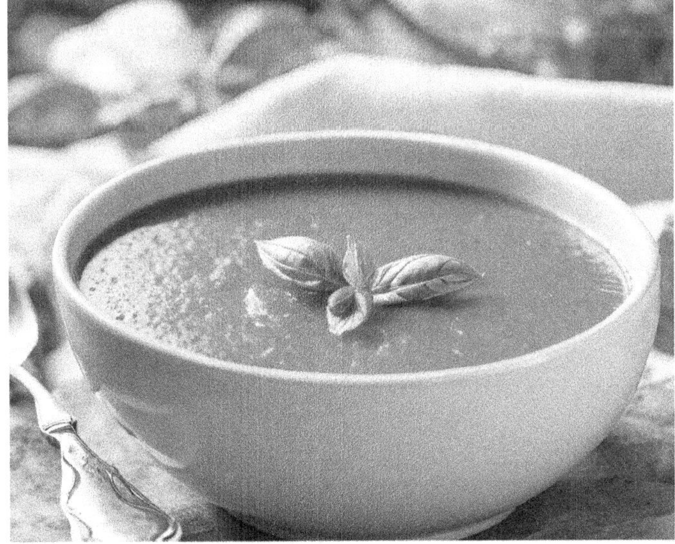

6. Spinach and Mushroom Soup

Ingredients:

- 1 tablespoon olive oil
- 1 large onion, chopped
- 2 cloves garlic, minced
- 2 cups sliced mushrooms (any variety)
- 4 cups low-sodium vegetable broth
- 4 cups fresh spinach, chopped
- 1/2 teaspoon thyme
- 1/2 teaspoon paprika
- 1/2 cup unsweetened almond milk

Instructions:

1. Heat the olive oil in a large pot over medium heat.
2. Add the chopped onion and cook until translucent, about 5 minutes.
3. Add the garlic and sliced mushrooms, cooking until the mushrooms are tender, about 5-7 minutes.
4. Stir in the vegetable broth, chopped spinach, thyme, and paprika. Bring to a boil.
5. Reduce heat and simmer for 15 minutes.
6. Stir in the almond milk and cook for an additional 5 minutes.
7. Serve hot.

Nutrition Info (per serving):

- Calories: 100
- Protein: 4g
- Carbohydrates: 12g
- Fiber: 3g
- Sugars: 3g
- Fat: 4g
- Saturated Fat: 0.5g

Serves: 4
Cooking Time: 30 minutes

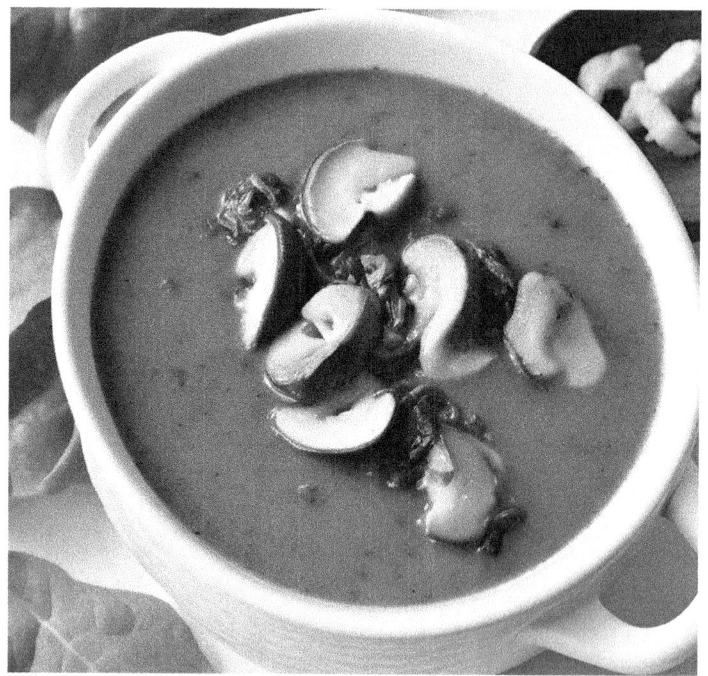

7. Zucchini Basil Soup

Ingredients:

- 1 tablespoon olive oil
- 1 large onion, chopped
- 2 cloves garlic, minced
- 4 cups chopped zucchini
- 4 cups low-sodium vegetable broth
- 1/2 cup chopped fresh basil
- 1 teaspoon dried oregano
- 1/2 cup unsweetened almond milk

Instructions:

1. Heat the olive oil in a large pot over medium heat.
2. Add the chopped onion and cook until translucent, about 5 minutes.
3. Add the garlic and chopped zucchini, cooking until the zucchini is tender, about 10 minutes.
4. Stir in the vegetable broth, fresh basil, and dried oregano. Bring to a boil.
5. Reduce heat and simmer for 15 minutes.
6. Use an immersion blender to puree the soup until smooth, or carefully transfer to a blender in batches and blend until smooth.
7. Stir in the almond milk and cook for an additional 5 minutes.
8. Serve hot.

Nutrition Info (per serving):

- Calories: 90
- Protein: 3g
- Carbohydrates: 12g
- Fiber: 3g
- Sugars: 4g
- Fat: 4g
- Saturated Fat: 0.5g

Serves: 4

Cooking Time: 30 minutes

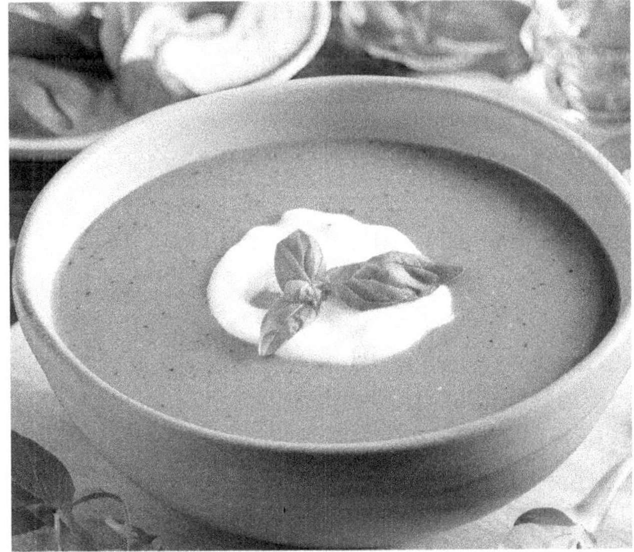

8. Garlic Roasted Brussels Sprouts

Ingredients:

- 1 pound Brussels sprouts, trimmed and halved
- 3 tablespoons olive oil
- 4 cloves garlic, minced
- 1 teaspoon dried thyme
- 1 tablespoon lemon juice

Instructions:

1. Preheat the oven to 400°F (200°C).
2. In a large bowl, toss the Brussels sprouts with the olive oil, minced garlic, and dried thyme.
3. Spread the Brussels sprouts on a baking sheet in a single layer.
4. Roast in the preheated oven for 20-25 minutes, until golden brown and crispy.
5. Drizzle with lemon juice before serving.
6. Serve hot.

Nutrition Info (per serving):

Calories: 140   Protein: 3g Carbohydrates: 10g   Fiber: 4g   Sugars: 2g Fat: 10g Saturated Fat: 1.5g

Serves: 4

Cooking Time: 30 minutes

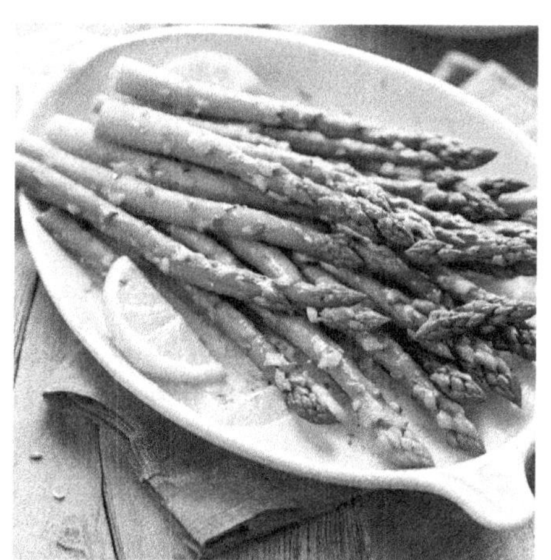

9. Grilled Asparagus with Lemon

Ingredients:

- 1 pound asparagus, trimmed
- 2 tablespoons olive oil
- 1 tablespoon lemon juice
- 1 teaspoon dried oregano

Instructions:

1. Preheat the grill to medium-high heat.
2. In a large bowl, toss the asparagus with the olive oil, lemon juice, and dried oregano.
3. Place the asparagus on the grill and cook for 5-7 minutes, turning occasionally, until tender and slightly charred.
4. Serve hot.

Nutrition Info (per serving):

Calories: 80 Protein: 2g Carbohydrates: 5g Fiber: 2g Sugars: 2g

- Fat: 7g
- Saturated Fat: 1g

Serves: 4

Cooking Time: 10 minutes

10. Balsamic Glazed Carrots

Ingredients:

- 1 pound carrots, peeled and sliced
- 2 tablespoons olive oil
- 2 tablespoons balsamic vinegar
- 1 tablespoon honey or maple syrup
- 1/2 teaspoon thyme

Instructions:

1. Preheat the oven to 400°F (200°C).
2. In a large bowl, toss the carrots with the olive oil, balsamic vinegar, honey or maple syrup, and thyme.
3. Spread the carrots on a baking sheet in a single layer.
4. Roast in the preheated oven for 20-25 minutes, until tender and caramelized.
5. Serve hot.

Nutrition Info (per serving):

- Calories: 120 Protein: 1g Carbohydrates: 15g Fiber: 3g Sugars: 9g
- Fat: 7g
- Saturated Fat: 1g

Serves: 4
Cooking Time: 30 minute

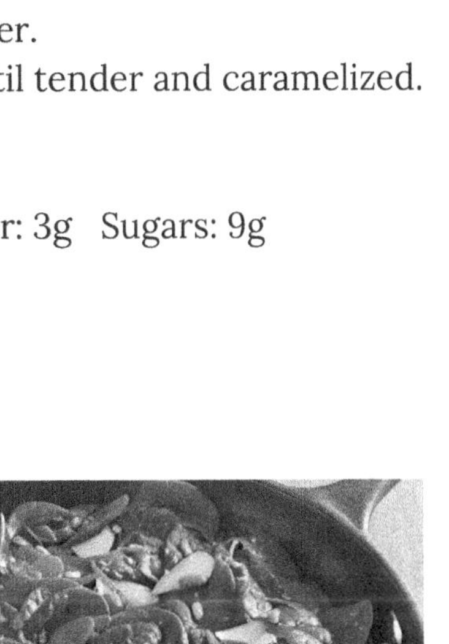

11. Garlic Spinach Sauté

Ingredients:

- 2 tablespoons olive oil
- 4 cloves garlic, minced
- 8 cups fresh spinach
- 1 tablespoon lemon juice
- 1/2 teaspoon paprika

Instructions:

1. Heat the olive oil in a large skillet over medium heat.
2. Add the minced garlic and cook for 1-2 minutes until fragrant.
3. Add the spinach to the skillet, stirring frequently until wilted, about 3-4 minutes.
4. Stir in the lemon juice and paprika.
5. Serve immediately.

Nutrition Info (per serving):

- Calories: 80 Protein: 2g Carbohydrates: 4g Fiber: 2g Sugars: 0g
- Fat: 7g
- Saturated Fat: 1g

Serves: 4
Cooking Time: 10 minutes

12. Mushroom and Green Bean Stir-Fry

Ingredients:

- 2 tablespoons olive oil
- 1 large onion, sliced
- 3 cloves garlic, minced
- 2 cups sliced mushrooms (any variety)
- 2 cups green beans, trimmed
- 2 tablespoons low-sodium soy sauce
- 1 tablespoon sesame seeds
- 1 tablespoon lemon juice

Instructions:

1. Heat the olive oil in a large skillet or wok over medium-high heat.
2. Add the sliced onion and cook for 3-4 minutes until softened.
3. Add the garlic and cook for another minute until fragrant.
4. Add the sliced mushrooms and green beans, stirring frequently, until the vegetables are tender, about 8-10 minutes.
5. Stir in the soy sauce, sesame seeds, and lemon juice.
6. Serve immediately.

Nutrition Info (per serving):

- Calories: 120
- Protein: 3g
- Carbohydrates: 10g
- Fiber: 4g
- Sugars: 4g
- Fat: 8g
- Saturated Fat: 1g

Serves: 4
Cooking Time: 15 minutes

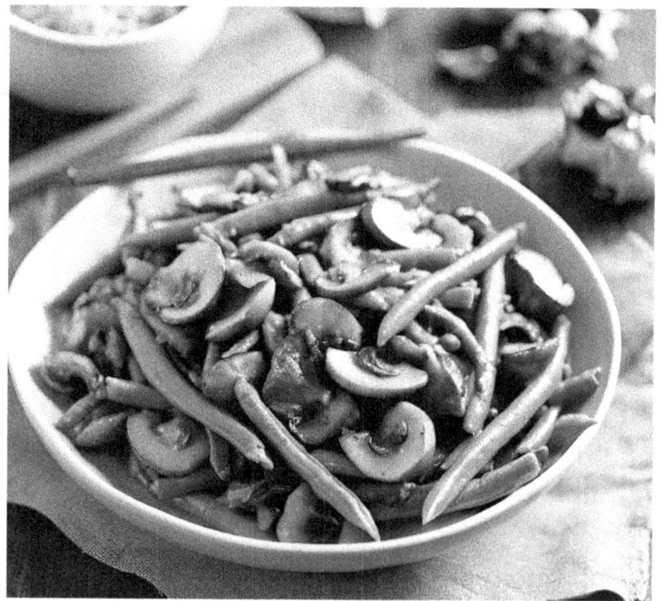

13. Bell Pepper and Tofu Stir-Fry

Ingredients:

- 2 tablespoons olive oil
- 1 block firm tofu, drained and cubed
- 1 red bell pepper, sliced
- 1 yellow bell pepper, sliced
- 1 green bell pepper, sliced
- 3 cloves garlic, minced
- 2 tablespoons low-sodium soy sauce
- 1 tablespoon rice vinegar
- 1 teaspoon ginger powder
- 1 tablespoon sesame seeds

Instructions:

1. Heat 1 tablespoon of olive oil in a large skillet or wok over medium-high heat.
2. Add the cubed tofu and cook until golden brown on all sides, about 5-7 minutes. Remove from the skillet and set aside.
3. Add the remaining olive oil to the skillet. Add the sliced bell peppers and garlic, cooking until tender, about 5-7 minutes.
4. Stir in the soy sauce, rice vinegar, and ginger powder. Cook for another 2-3 minutes.
5. Return the tofu to the skillet and toss to combine.
6. Sprinkle with sesame seeds and serve immediately.

Nutrition Info (per serving):

- Calories: 180
- Protcin: 9g
- Carbohydrates: 12g
- Fiber: 4g
- Sugars: 5g
- Fat: 12g
- Saturated Fat: 2g

Serves: 4
Cooking Time: 20 minutes

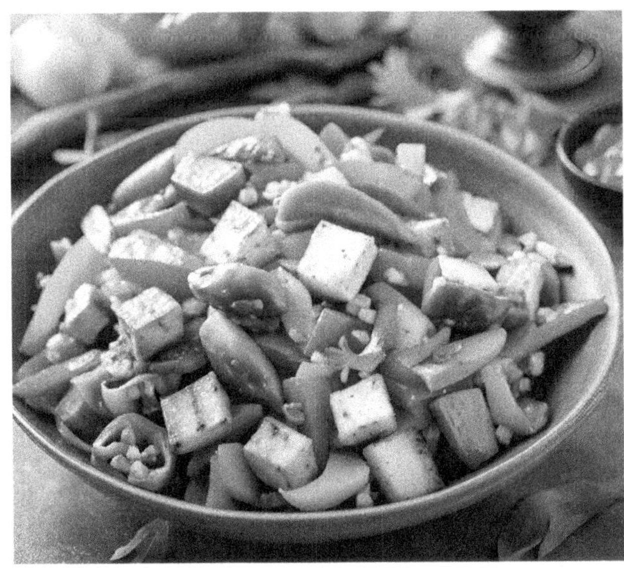

14. Eggplant and Tomato Stir-Fry

Ingredients:

- 2 tablespoons olive oil
- 1 large eggplant, cubed
- 1 large onion, chopped
- 3 cloves garlic, minced
- 2 cups cherry tomatoes, halved
- 1 teaspoon dried oregano
- 1 tablespoon balsamic vinegar

Instructions:

1. Heat the olive oil in a large skillet or wok over medium-high heat.
2. Add the cubed eggplant and cook until tender and golden brown, about 8-10 minutes.
3. Add the chopped onion and cook for another 3-4 minutes until softened.
4. Add the garlic and cherry tomatoes, cooking until the tomatoes start to soften, about 3-4 minutes.
5. Stir in the dried oregano and balsamic vinegar. Cook for another 2-3 minutes.
6. Serve immediately.

Nutrition Info (per serving):

- Calories: 140
- Protein: 2g
- Carbohydrates: 14g
- Fiber: 5g
- Sugars: 8g
- Fat: 9g
- Saturated Fat: 1.5g

Serves: 4
Cooking Time: 20 minutes

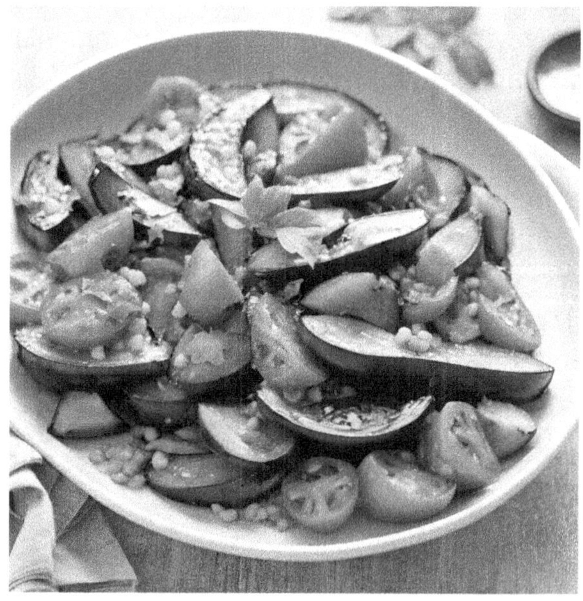

15. Zucchini and Corn Stir-Fry

Ingredients:

- 2 tablespoons olive oil
- 1 large onion, chopped
- 2 cloves garlic, minced
- 2 medium zucchinis, sliced
- 1 cup fresh or frozen corn kernels
- 1 teaspoon dried basil
- 1 tablespoon lemon juice

Instructions:

1. Heat the olive oil in a large skillet or wok over medium-high heat.
2. Add the chopped onion and cook until translucent, about 5 minutes.
3. Add the garlic and cook for another minute until fragrant.
4. Add the sliced zucchinis and cook until tender, about 5-7 minutes.
5. Stir in the corn kernels and dried basil, cooking for another 3-4 minutes.
6. Stir in the lemon juice before serving.
7. Serve immediately.

Nutrition Info (per serving):

- Calories: 120
- Protein: 2g
- Carbohydrates: 15g
- Fiber: 3g
- Sugars: 5g
- Fat: 7g
- Saturated Fat: 1g

Serves: 4

Cooking Time: 15 minutes

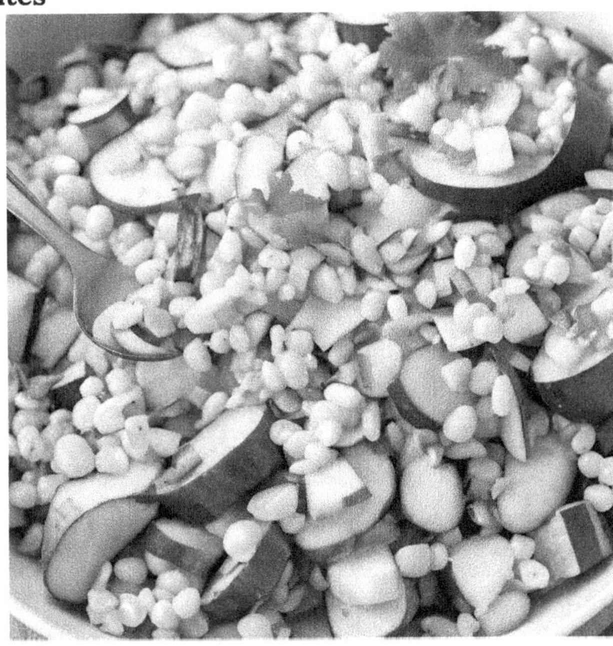

16. Acorn Squash with Quinoa

Ingredients:

- 2 acorn squashes, halved and seeds removed
- 1 cup quinoa
- 2 cups low-sodium vegetable broth
- 1/2 cup dried cranberries (unsweetened)
- 1/4 cup chopped walnuts
- 1 tablespoon olive oil
- 1 teaspoon ground cumin
- 1/2 teaspoon paprika
- 1 tablespoon honey or maple syrup

Instructions:

1. Preheat the oven to 375°F (190°C).
2. Place the acorn squash halves cut side up on a baking sheet. Brush with olive oil and roast in the preheated oven for 35-40 minutes, until tender.
3. While the squash is roasting, rinse the quinoa under cold water. In a medium saucepan, bring the vegetable broth to a boil.
4. Add the quinoa, reduce heat, and simmer for 15 minutes, until the broth is absorbed and the quinoa is tender.
5. In a large bowl, combine the cooked quinoa, dried cranberries, chopped walnuts, ground cumin, paprika, and honey or maple syrup.
6. Once the squash is done roasting, fill each half with the quinoa mixture.
7. Serve immediately.

Nutrition Info (per serving):

- Calories: 250
- Protein: 6g
- Carbohydrates: 45g
- Fiber: 6g
- Sugars: 12g
- Fat: 8g
- Saturated Fat: 1g

Serves: 4
Cooking Time: 40 minutes

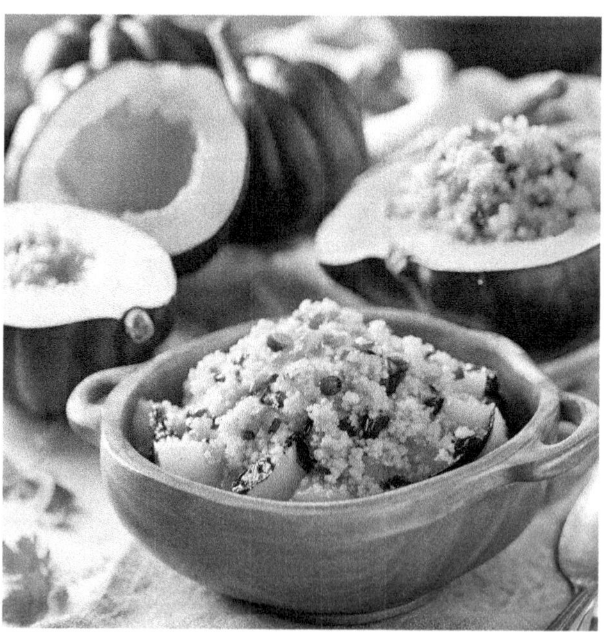

17. Baked Tomatoes with Pesto

Ingredients:

- 4 large tomatoes
- 1/2 cup homemade or store-bought pesto (without cheese for a vegan option)
- 1/4 cup whole grain breadcrumbs
- 2 tablespoons olive oil
- 1/4 cup chopped fresh basil

Instructions:

1. Preheat the oven to 375°F (190°C).
2. Cut the tops off the tomatoes and scoop out the seeds and pulp.
3. Fill each tomato with 2 tablespoons of pesto.
4. In a small bowl, mix the breadcrumbs with olive oil until evenly coated.
5. Sprinkle the breadcrumb mixture over the top of each stuffed tomato.
6. Place the tomatoes in a baking dish and bake in the preheated oven for 20-25 minutes, until the tomatoes are tender and the breadcrumbs are golden brown.
7. Garnish with chopped fresh basil and serve immediately.

Nutrition Info (per serving):

- Calories: 160
- Protein: 3g
- Carbohydrates: 12g
- Fiber: 3g
- Sugars: 5g
- Fat: 12g
- Saturated Fat: 1.5g

Servcs: 4
Cooking Time: 25 minutes

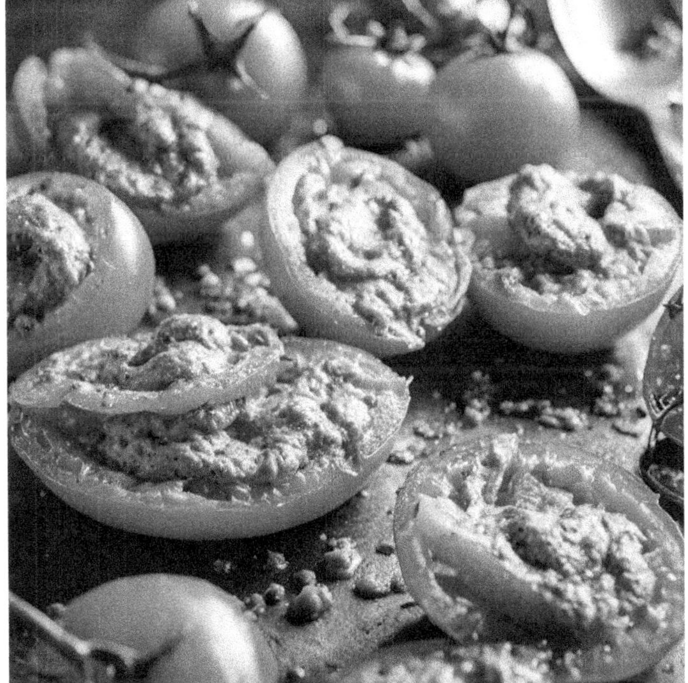

18. Stuffed Portobello Mushrooms

Ingredients:

- 4 large portobello mushrooms
- 1 cup cooked quinoa
- 1/2 cup chopped spinach
- 1/4 cup sun-dried tomatoes (not in oil), chopped
- 2 tablespoons olive oil
- 2 cloves garlic, minced
- 1 teaspoon dried oregano
- 1/4 cup nutritional yeast (optional)

Instructions:

1. Preheat the oven to 375°F (190°C).
2. Clean the portobello mushrooms and remove the stems. Place them on a baking sheet.
3. In a large skillet, heat the olive oil over medium heat. Add the minced garlic and cook for 1 minute until fragrant.
4. Add the chopped spinach and sun-dried tomatoes, cooking until the spinach is wilted, about 3-4 minutes.
5. In a large bowl, combine the cooked quinoa, spinach mixture, dried oregano, and nutritional yeast (if using).
6. Fill each portobello mushroom with the quinoa mixture.
7. Bake in the preheated oven for 20-25 minutes, until the mushrooms are tender.
8. Serve immediately.

Nutrition Info (per serving):

- Calories: 180
- Protein: 7g
- Carbohydrates: 20g
- Fiber: 4g
- Sugars: 4g
- Fat: 8g
- Saturated Fat: 1g

Serves: 4

Cooking Time: 25 minutes

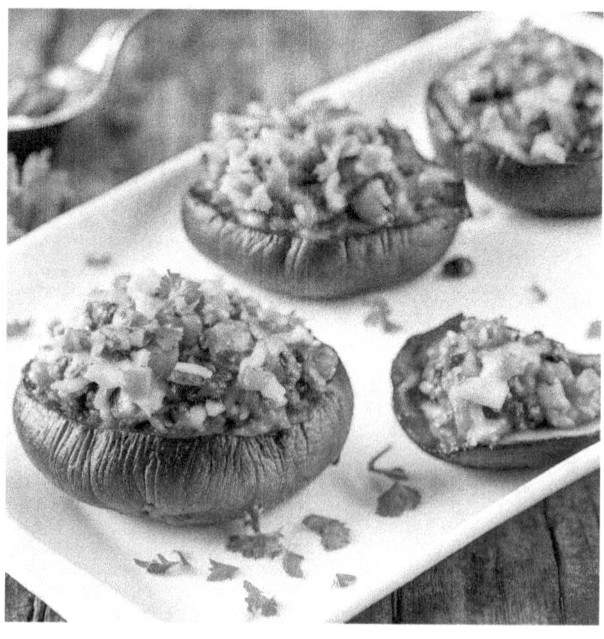

19. Sweet Potatoes Stuffed with Kale

Ingredients:

- 4 medium sweet potatoes
- 1 tablespoon olive oil
- 1 small onion, chopped
- 2 cloves garlic, minced
- 4 cups chopped kale (stems removed)
- 1/2 teaspoon ground cumin
- 1/4 teaspoon paprika
- 1/4 cup chopped walnuts
- 1 tablespoon lemon juice

Instructions:

1. Preheat the oven to 400°F (200°C).
2. Pierce the sweet potatoes with a fork and bake in the preheated oven for 45-50 minutes, until tender.
3. While the sweet potatoes are baking, heat the olive oil in a large skillet over medium heat. Add the chopped onion and cook until translucent, about 5 minutes.
4. Add the minced garlic and cook for another minute.
5. Add the chopped kale, ground cumin, and paprika, cooking until the kale is wilted, about 5-7 minutes.
6. Stir in the chopped walnuts and lemon juice.
7. Once the sweet potatoes are done, slice them open and fill each with the kale mixture.
8. Serve immediately.

Nutrition Info (per serving):

- Calories: 250
- Protein: 5g
- Carbohydrates: 40g
- Fiber: 7g
- Sugars: 10g
- Fat: 10g
- Saturated Fat: 1.5g

Serves: 4

Cooking Time: 50 minutes

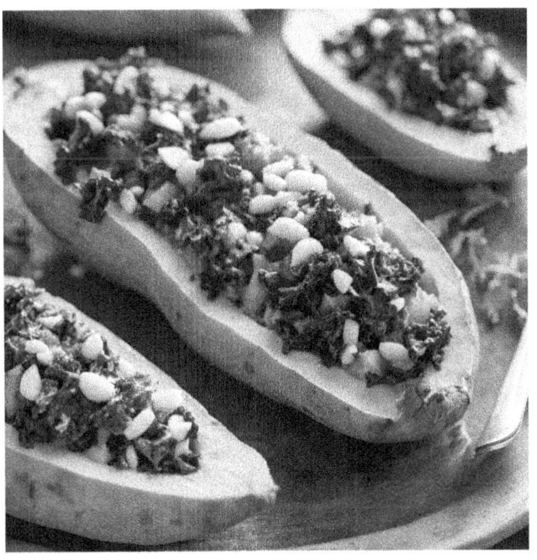

20. Vegetable Lasagna

Ingredients:

- 9 whole grain lasagna noodles
- 2 tablespoons olive oil
- 1 large onion, chopped
- 3 cloves garlic, minced
- 2 cups sliced mushrooms
- 2 cups chopped spinach
- 2 cups chopped zucchini
- 1 cup shredded carrots
- 2 cups low-fat ricotta cheese
- 1/2 cup grated Parmesan cheese
- 2 cups marinara sauce (low sodium)
- 1 cup shredded mozzarella cheese

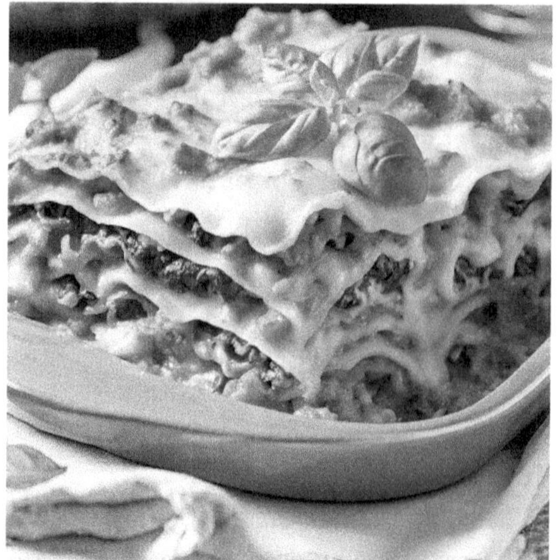

Instructions:

1. Preheat the oven to 375°F (190°C).
2. Cook the lasagna noodles according to package instructions. Drain and set aside.
3. In a large skillet, heat the olive oil over medium heat. Add the chopped onion and cook until translucent, about 5 minutes.
4. Add the garlic and mushrooms, cooking until the mushrooms are tender, about 5 minutes.
5. Add the spinach, zucchini, and shredded carrots, cooking until the vegetables are tender, about 5-7 minutes.
6. In a medium bowl, combine the ricotta cheese and grated Parmesan cheese.
7. Spread 1/2 cup of marinara sauce on the bottom of a 9x13-inch baking dish.
8. Place 3 lasagna noodles over the sauce. Spread 1/3 of the ricotta mixture over the noodles. Top with 1/3 of the vegetable mixture and 1/2 cup of marinara sauce.
9. Repeat the layers two more times, ending with a layer of marinara sauce.
10. Sprinkle the shredded mozzarella cheese on top.
11. Cover with aluminum foil and bake for 30 minutes. Remove the foil and bake for an additional 10 minutes, until the cheese is golden and bubbly.
12. Let the lasagna sit for 10 minutes before serving.

Nutrition Info (per serving):

- Calories: 320
- Protein: 16g
- Carbohydrates: 40g
- Fiber: 7g
- Sugars: 9g
- Fat: 12g
- Saturated Fat: 5g

Serves: 6

Cooking Time: 60 minutes

21. Cauliflower Gratin

Ingredients:

- 1 large cauliflower, cut into florets
- 2 tablespoons olive oil
- 1 large onion, chopped
- 2 cloves garlic, minced
- 1 cup unsweetened almond milk
- 1/2 cup low-fat Greek yogurt
- 1/4 cup grated Parmesan cheese
- 1 teaspoon thyme
- 1/4 teaspoon nutmeg
- 1/2 cup whole grain breadcrumbs

Instructions:

1. Preheat the oven to 375°F (190°C).
2. Steam the cauliflower florets until tender, about 10 minutes. Drain and set aside.
3. In a large skillet, heat the olive oil over medium heat. Add the chopped onion and cook until translucent, about 5 minutes.
4. Add the garlic and cook for another minute.
5. In a large bowl, combine the steamed cauliflower, cooked onion and garlic, almond milk, Greek yogurt, Parmesan cheese, thyme, and nutmeg. Mix well.
6. Transfer the mixture to a 9x13-inch baking dish.
7. Sprinkle the whole grain breadcrumbs on top.
8. Bake in the preheated oven for 25-30 minutes, until the top is golden brown.
9. Serve hot.

Nutrition Info (per serving):

- Calories: 160
- Protein: 6g
- Carbohydrates: 16g
- Fiber: 4g
- Sugars: 5g
- Fat: 9g
- Saturated Fat: 2g

Serves: 6
Cooking Time: 40 minutes

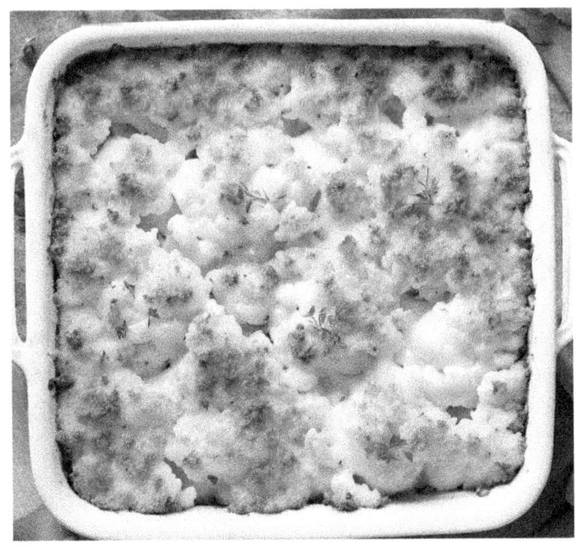

22. Greek Stuffed Eggplant

Ingredients:

- 2 large eggplants, halved and scooped out
- 2 tablespoons olive oil
- 1 large onion, chopped
- 3 cloves garlic, minced
- 1 cup cooked quinoa
- 1/2 cup chopped tomatoes
- 1/4 cup chopped fresh parsley
- 1 teaspoon dried oregano
- 1/4 cup crumbled feta cheese

Instructions:

1. Preheat the oven to 375°F (190°C).
2. Place the eggplant halves in a baking dish and bake for 20 minutes, until tender.
3. In a large skillet, heat the olive oil over medium heat. Add the chopped onion and cook until translucent, about 5 minutes.
4. Add the garlic and cook for another minute.
5. Add the scooped-out eggplant flesh, chopped tomatoes, and dried oregano. Cook until the vegetables are tender, about 5-7 minutes.
6. Stir in the cooked quinoa and chopped parsley.
7. Remove the eggplant halves from the oven and fill each with the quinoa mixture.
8. Sprinkle the crumbled feta cheese on top.
9. Bake for an additional 10-15 minutes, until the cheese is melted.
10. Serve hot.

Nutrition Info (per serving):

- Calories: 200
- Protein: 7g
- Carbohydrates: 26g
- Fiber: 7g
- Sugars: 10g
- Fat: 9g
- Saturated Fat: 2g

Serves: 4

Cooking Time: 40 minutes

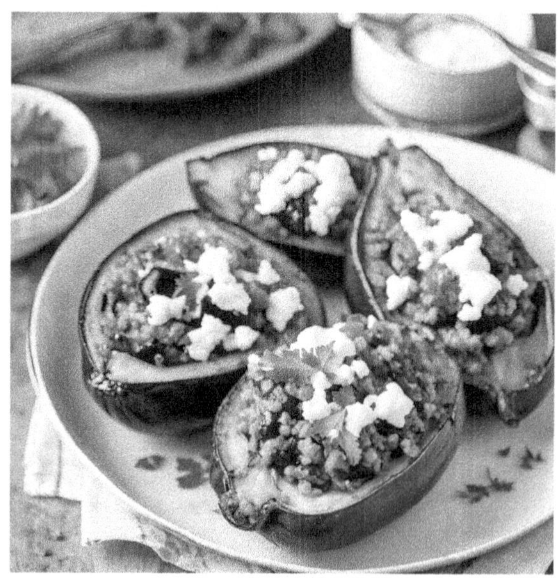

23. Moroccan Vegetable Tagine

Ingredients:

- 2 tablespoons olive oil
- 1 large onion, chopped
- 3 cloves garlic, minced
- 2 cups chopped carrots
- 2 cups chopped zucchini
- 1 cup chickpeas, rinsed and drained
- 1 cup chopped tomatoes
- 1/2 cup dried apricots, chopped
- 2 teaspoons ground cumin
- 1 teaspoon ground cinnamon
- 1 teaspoon ground ginger
- 2 cups low-sodium vegetable broth
- 1/4 cup chopped fresh cilantro

Instructions:

1. Heat the olive oil in a large pot or Dutch oven over medium heat.
2. Add the chopped onion and cook until translucent, about 5 minutes.
3. Add the garlic and cook for another minute.
4. Stir in the chopped carrots, zucchini, chickpeas, tomatoes, and dried apricots.
5. Add the ground cumin, cinnamon, and ginger, cooking for 1-2 minutes until fragrant.
6. Pour in the vegetable broth and bring to a boil.
7. Reduce heat and simmer for 25-30 minutes, until the vegetables are tender.
8. Stir in the chopped fresh cilantro before serving.
9. Serve hot.

Nutrition Info (per serving):

- Calories: 250
- Protein: 6g
- Carbohydrates: 42g
- Fiber: 9g
- Sugars: 18g
- Fat: 7g
- Saturated Fat: 1g

Serves: 4

Cooking Time: 45 minutes

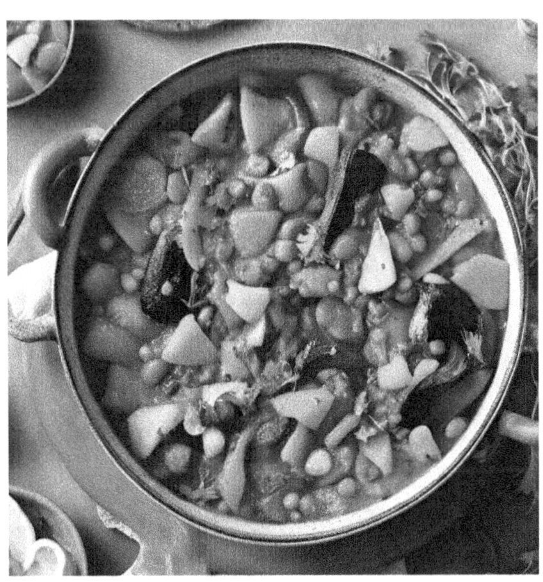

24. Japanese Miso Eggplant

Ingredients:

- 4 small eggplants, halved
- 2 tablespoons olive oil
- 1/4 cup miso paste
- 2 tablespoons rice vinegar
- 2 tablespoons mirin (sweet rice wine)
- 1 tablespoon sesame oil
- 1 tablespoon honey or maple syrup
- 2 green onions, chopped

Instructions:

1. Preheat the oven to 400°F (200°C).
2. Score the flesh of the eggplant halves and place them on a baking sheet. Brush with olive oil.
3. Roast in the preheated oven for 20-25 minutes, until tender.
4. In a small bowl, whisk together the miso paste, rice vinegar, mirin, sesame oil, and honey or maple syrup.
5. Remove the eggplants from the oven and brush with the miso mixture.
6. Return to the oven and bake for an additional 5-7 minutes.
7. Sprinkle with chopped green onions before serving.
8. Serve hot.

Nutrition Info (per serving):

- Calories: 180
- Protein: 3g
- Carbohydrates: 16g
- Fiber: 4g
- Sugars: 8g
- Fat: 12g
- Saturated Fat: 2g

Serves: 4

Cooking Time: 35 minutes

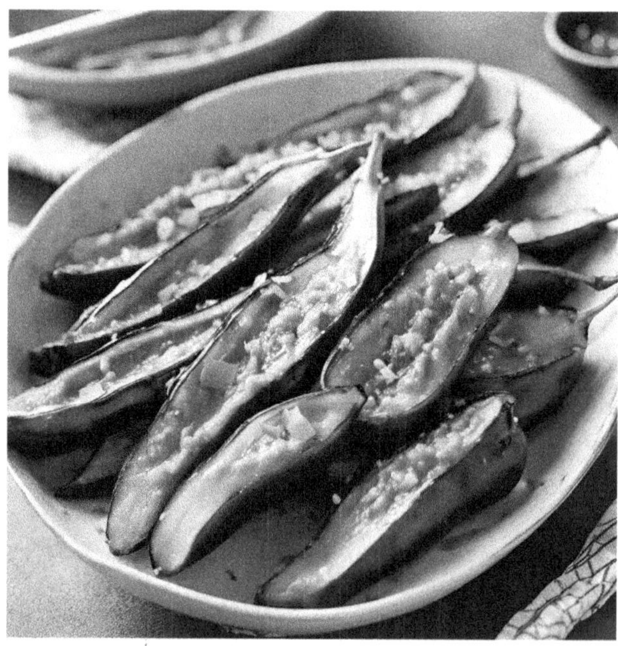

25. Vegetable Nori Rolls

Ingredients:

- 4 nori sheets
- 2 cups cooked brown rice
- 1 avocado, sliced
- 1 cucumber, julienned
- 1 carrot, julienned
- 1/4 cup shredded red cabbage
- 2 tablespoons rice vinegar
- 1 tablespoon sesame seeds

Instructions:

1. In a small bowl, mix the cooked brown rice with rice vinegar.
2. Place a nori sheet on a bamboo sushi mat, shiny side down.
3. Spread 1/2 cup of the rice mixture evenly over the nori sheet, leaving a 1-inch border at the top.
4. Arrange avocado slices, cucumber, carrot, and shredded red cabbage in a line along the bottom edge of the rice.
5. Roll the nori tightly from the bottom, using the bamboo mat to help.
6. Seal the edge with a little water.
7. Slice the roll into 6-8 pieces and sprinkle with sesame seeds.
8. Repeat with the remaining nori sheets.
9. Serve immediately.

Nutrition Info (per serving):

- Calories: 150
- Protcin: 4g
- Carbohydrates: 24g
- Fibcr: 5g
- Sugars: 2g
- Fat: 6g
- Saturated Fat: 1g

Serves: 4
Cooking Time: 20 minutes

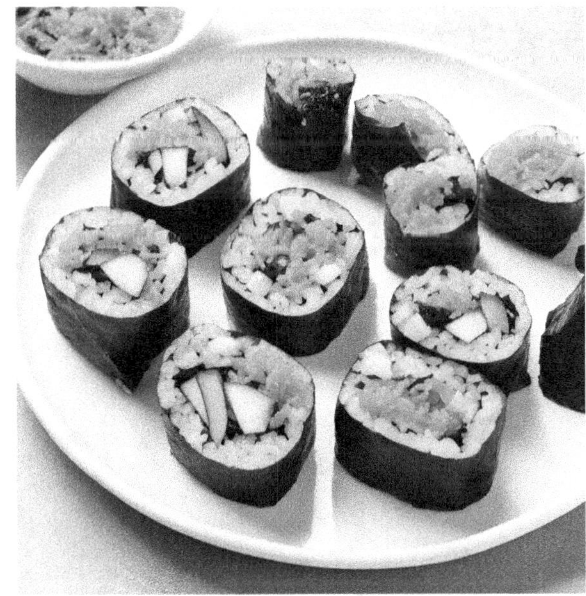

26. Zucchini Noodles with Pesto

Ingredients:

- 4 medium zucchinis, spiralized
- 1/4 cup homemade or store-bought pesto (without cheese for a vegan option)
- 1 tablespoon olive oil
- 1/4 cup chopped cherry tomatoes
- 2 tablespoons pine nuts

Instructions:

1. Heat the olive oil in a large skillet over medium heat.
2. Add the spiralized zucchini noodles and cook for 3-4 minutes, until just tender.
3. Remove from heat and toss with pesto.
4. Stir in the chopped cherry tomatoes.
5. Serve immediately, topped with pine nuts.

Nutrition Info (per serving):

- Calories: 180
- Protein: 4g
- Carbohydrates: 10g
- Fiber: 3g
- Sugars: 6g
- Fat: 15g
- Saturated Fat: 2g

Serves: 4
Cooking Time: 10 minutes

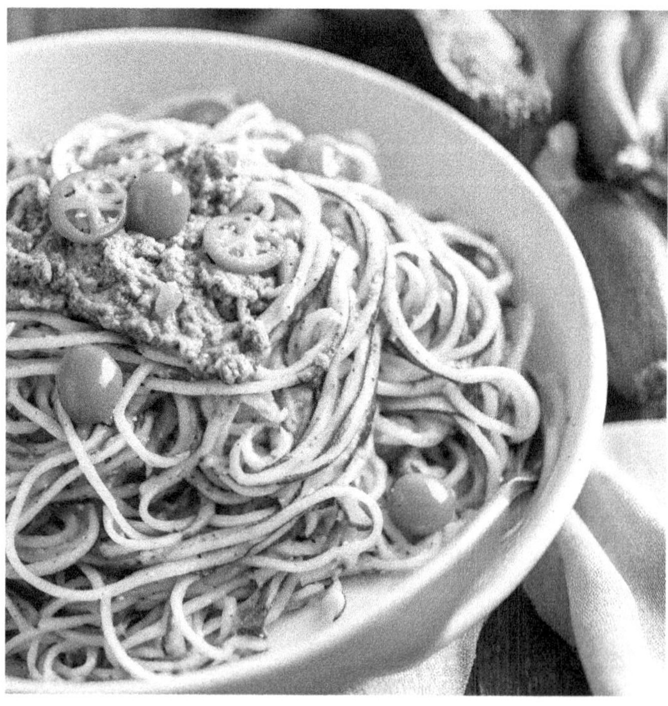

Soup and Stew Recipes

1. Spinach and White Bean Soup

Ingredients:
- 2 tablespoons olive oil
- 1 large onion, chopped
- 3 cloves garlic, minced
- 4 cups low-sodium vegetable broth
- 2 cans (15 oz each) white beans, rinsed and drained
- 4 cups fresh spinach, chopped
- 1 teaspoon dried thyme
- 1 teaspoon paprika
- 1 tablespoon lemon juice

Instructions:
1. Heat the olive oil in a large pot over medium heat.
2. Add the chopped onion and cook until translucent, about 5 minutes.
3. Add the garlic and cook for another minute until fragrant.
4. Pour in the vegetable broth and add the white beans, thyme, and paprika. Bring to a boil.
5. Reduce heat and simmer for 15 minutes.
6. Stir in the chopped spinach and cook until wilted, about 3-4 minutes.
7. Add the lemon juice and stir well.
8. Serve hot.

Nutrition Info (per serving):
- Calories: 180
- Protein: 8g
- Carbohydrates: 24g
- Fiber: 8g
- Sugars: 2g
- Fat: 6g
- Saturated Fat: 1g

Serves: 4

Cooking Time: 30 minutes

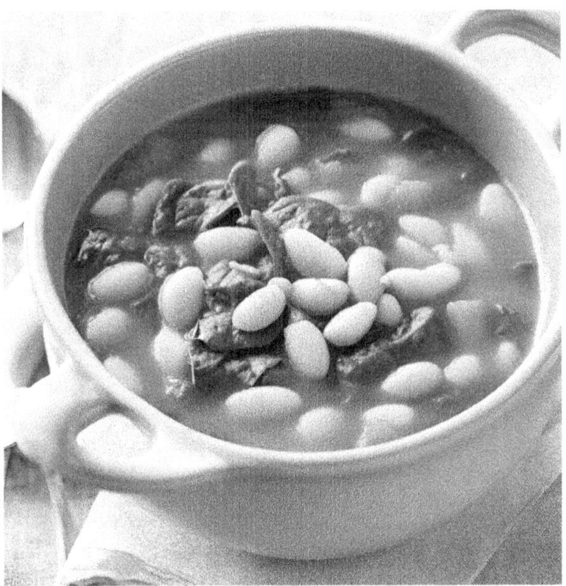

2. Sweet Potato and Lentil Soup

Ingredients:

- 2 tablespoons olive oil
- 1 large onion, chopped
- 2 cloves garlic, minced
- 2 cups diced sweet potatoes
- 1 cup red lentils, rinsed
- 4 cups low-sodium vegetable broth
- 1 teaspoon ground cumin
- 1/2 teaspoon ground turmeric
- 1/2 teaspoon paprika
- 1 tablespoon lemon juice

Instructions:

1. Heat the olive oil in a large pot over medium heat.
2. Add the chopped onion and cook until translucent, about 5 minutes.
3. Add the garlic and cook for another minute until fragrant.
4. Stir in the diced sweet potatoes and red lentils.
5. Pour in the vegetable broth and add the cumin, turmeric, and paprika. Bring to a boil.
6. Reduce heat and simmer for 25-30 minutes, until the sweet potatoes and lentils are tender.
7. Stir in the lemon juice.
8. Serve hot.

Nutrition Info (per serving):

- Calories: 220
- Protein: 8g
- Carbohydrates: 35g
- Fiber: 10g
- Sugars: 6g
- Fat: 6g
- Saturated Fat: 1g

Serves: 4

Cooking Time: 35 minutes

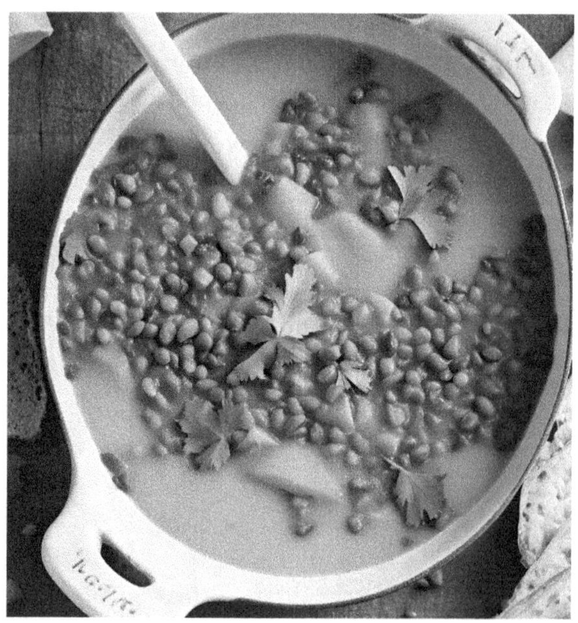

3. Fennel and Potato Soup

Ingredients:

- 2 tablespoons olive oil
- 1 large onion, chopped
- 2 cloves garlic, minced
- 2 bulbs fennel, trimmed and sliced
- 4 cups diced potatoes
- 4 cups low-sodium vegetable broth
- 1 teaspoon dried thyme
- 1/2 teaspoon paprika
- 1 tablespoon lemon juice

Instructions:

1. Heat the olive oil in a large pot over medium heat.
2. Add the chopped onion and cook until translucent, about 5 minutes.
3. Add the garlic and sliced fennel, cooking until the fennel is tender, about 5-7 minutes.
4. Stir in the diced potatoes.
5. Pour in the vegetable broth and add the thyme and paprika. Bring to a boil.
6. Reduce heat and simmer for 25-30 minutes, until the potatoes are tender.
7. Use an immersion blender to puree the soup until smooth, or carefully transfer to a blender in batches and blend until smooth.
8. Stir in the lemon juice.
9. Serve hot.

Nutrition Info (per serving):

- Calories: 200
- Protein: 4g
- Carbohydrates: 30g
- Fiber: 6g
- Sugars: 5g
- Fat: 7g
- Saturated Fat: 1g

Serves: 4
Cooking Time: 40 minutes

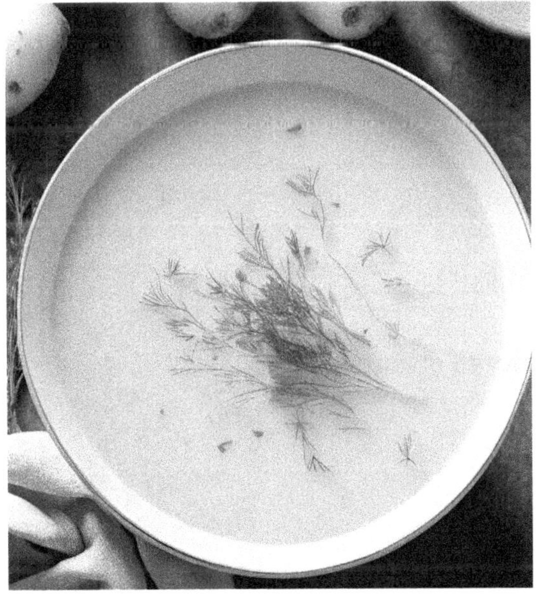

4. Eggplant and Chickpea Stew

Ingredients:

- 2 tablespoons olive oil
- 1 large onion, chopped
- 3 cloves garlic, minced
- 1 large eggplant, cubed
- 2 cups chopped tomatoes
- 1 can (15 oz) chickpeas, rinsed and drained
- 1 teaspoon ground cumin
- 1 teaspoon paprika
- 1 teaspoon dried oregano
- 4 cups low-sodium vegetable broth
- 1/4 cup chopped fresh parsley

Instructions:

1. Heat the olive oil in a large pot over medium heat.
2. Add the chopped onion and cook until translucent, about 5 minutes.
3. Add the garlic and cubed eggplant, cooking until the eggplant is tender, about 8-10 minutes.
4. Stir in the chopped tomatoes, chickpeas, cumin, paprika, and oregano.
5. Pour in the vegetable broth and bring to a boil.
6. Reduce heat and simmer for 25-30 minutes, until the stew is thickened.
7. Stir in the chopped parsley before serving.
8. Serve hot.

Nutrition Info (per serving):

- Calories: 220
- Protein: 6g
- Carbohydrates: 30g
- Fiber: 8g
- Sugars: 8g
- Fat: 10g
- Saturated Fat: 1.5g

Serves: 4

Cooking Time: 45 minutes

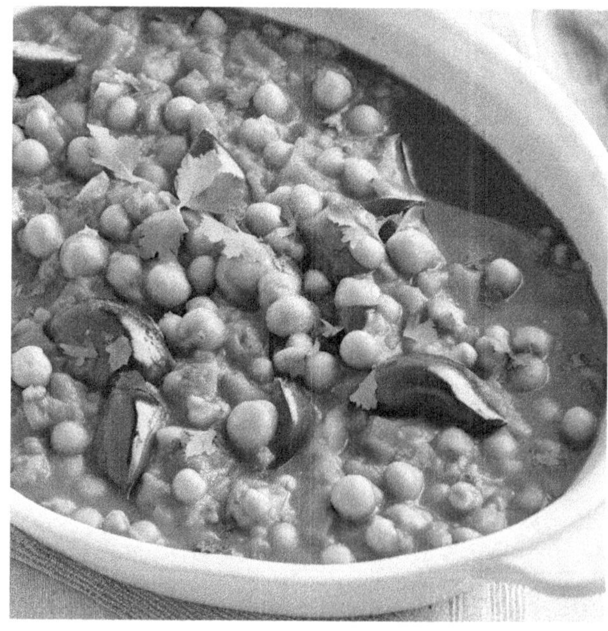

5. Kale and White Bean Stew

Ingredients:

- 2 tablespoons olive oil
- 1 large onion, chopped
- 3 cloves garlic, minced
- 4 cups chopped kale
- 2 cans (15 oz each) white beans, rinsed and drained
- 4 cups low-sodium vegetable broth
- 1 teaspoon dried thyme
- 1 teaspoon paprika
- 1 tablespoon lemon juice

Instructions:

1. Heat the olive oil in a large pot over medium heat.
2. Add the chopped onion and cook until translucent, about 5 minutes.
3. Add the garlic and chopped kale, cooking until the kale is wilted, about 5-7 minutes.
4. Stir in the white beans, vegetable broth, thyme, and paprika. Bring to a boil.
5. Reduce heat and simmer for 20 minutes.
6. Stir in the lemon juice before serving.
7. Serve hot.

Nutrition Info (per serving):

- Calories: 190
- Protein: 8g
- Carbohydrates: 28g
- Fiber: 9g
- Sugars: 3g
- Fat: 6g
- Saturated Fat: 1g

Serves: 4
Cooking Time: 30 minutes

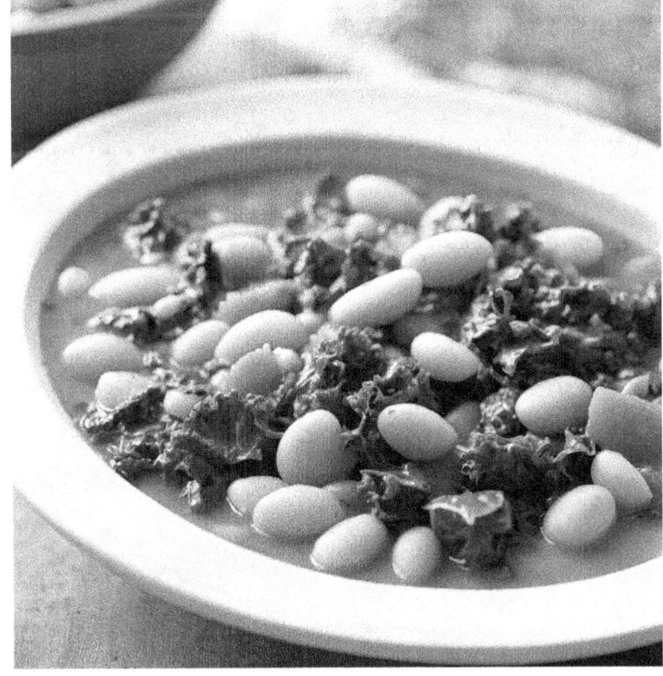

6. Zucchini and Tomato Stew

Ingredients:

- 2 tablespoons olive oil
- 1 large onion, chopped
- 2 cloves garlic, minced
- 4 cups chopped zucchini
- 2 cups chopped tomatoes
- 1 can (15 oz) chickpeas, rinsed and drained
- 1 teaspoon dried oregano
- 1 teaspoon ground cumin
- 1/2 teaspoon paprika
- 4 cups low-sodium vegetable broth
- 1/4 cup chopped fresh basil

Instructions:

1. Heat the olive oil in a large pot over medium heat.
2. Add the chopped onion and cook until translucent, about 5 minutes.
3. Add the garlic and chopped zucchini, cooking until the zucchini is tender, about 5-7 minutes.
4. Stir in the chopped tomatoes, chickpeas, oregano, cumin, and paprika.
5. Pour in the vegetable broth and bring to a boil.
6. Reduce heat and simmer for 25-30 minutes, until the stew is thickened.
7. Stir in the chopped fresh basil before serving.
8. Serve hot.

Nutrition Info (per serving):

- Calories: 180
- Protein: 6g
- Carbohydrates: 28g
- Fiber: 8g
- Sugars: 8g
- Fat: 6g
- Saturated Fat: 1g

Serves: 4

Cooking Time: 45 minutes

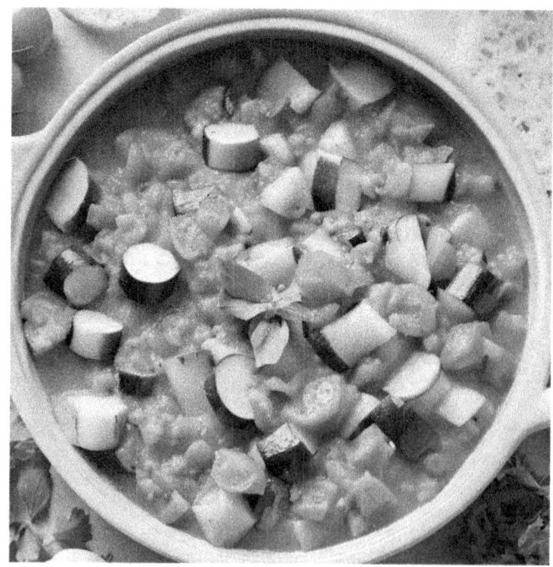

7. Okra and Tomato Stew

Ingredients:

- 2 tablespoons olive oil
- 1 large onion, chopped
- 3 cloves garlic, minced
- 4 cups sliced okra
- 2 cups chopped tomatoes
- 1 can (15 oz) chickpeas, rinsed and drained
- 1 teaspoon ground cumin
- 1 teaspoon paprika
- 4 cups low-sodium vegetable broth
- 1 tablespoon lemon juice
- 1/4 cup chopped fresh parsley

Instructions:

1. Heat the olive oil in a large pot over medium heat.
2. Add the chopped onion and cook until translucent, about 5 minutes.
3. Add the garlic and cook for another minute until fragrant.
4. Stir in the sliced okra and cook for 5-7 minutes until tender.
5. Add the chopped tomatoes, chickpeas, cumin, and paprika.
6. Pour in the vegetable broth and bring to a boil.
7. Reduce heat and simmer for 20-25 minutes until the stew is thickened.
8. Stir in the lemon juice and chopped fresh parsley before serving.
9. Serve hot.

Nutrition Info (per serving):

- Calories: 170
- Protein: 5g
- Carbohydrates: 24g
- Fiber: 8g
- Sugars: 6g
- Fat: 7g
- Saturated Fat: 1g

Serves: 4
Cooking Time: 35 minutes

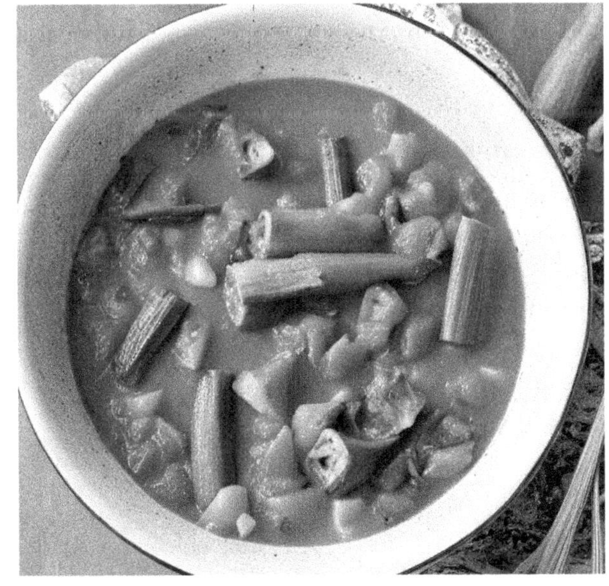

8. Brazilian Black Bean Stew

Ingredients:

- 2 tablespoons olive oil
- 1 large onion, chopped
- 3 cloves garlic, minced
- 1 red bell pepper, chopped
- 1 green bell pepper, chopped
- 2 cans (15 oz each) black beans, rinsed and drained
- 4 cups low-sodium vegetable broth
- 1 teaspoon ground cumin
- 1 teaspoon smoked paprika
- 1/2 teaspoon ground coriander
- 1/4 cup chopped fresh cilantro
- 1 tablespoon lime juice

Instructions:

1. Heat the olive oil in a large pot over medium heat.
2. Add the chopped onion and cook until translucent, about 5 minutes.
3. Add the garlic, red bell pepper, and green bell pepper, cooking until tender, about 5-7 minutes.
4. Stir in the black beans, vegetable broth, cumin, smoked paprika, and ground coriander. Bring to a boil.
5. Reduce heat and simmer for 25-30 minutes, until the stew is thickened.
6. Stir in the chopped fresh cilantro and lime juice before serving.
7. Serve hot.

Nutrition Info (per serving):

- Calories: 220
- Protein: 10g
- Carbohydrates: 34g
- Fiber: 12g
- Sugars: 6g
- Fat: 7g
- Saturated Fat: 1g

Serves: 4

Cooking Time: 40 minutes

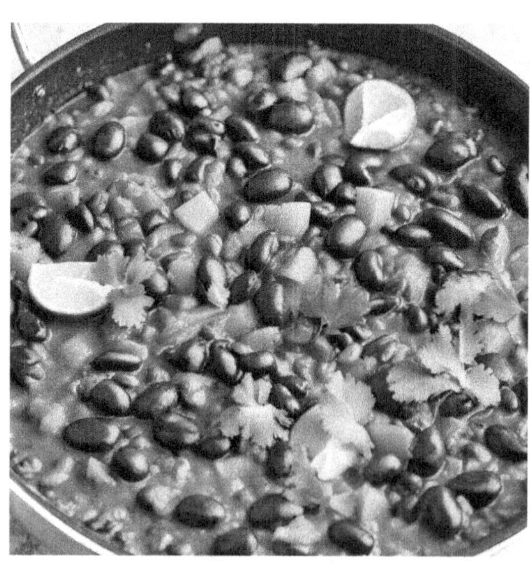

9. Asian Tofu and Vegetable Stew

Ingredients:
- 2 tablespoons sesame oil
- 1 large onion, chopped
- 3 cloves garlic, minced
- 1 tablespoon grated ginger
- 1 block firm tofu, cubed
- 2 cups chopped bok choy
- 1 cup sliced carrots
- 1 cup sliced mushrooms (shiitake or button)
- 4 cups low-sodium vegetable broth
- 2 tablespoons low-sodium soy sauce
- 1 tablespoon rice vinegar
- 1 tablespoon miso paste (optional)
- 1/4 cup chopped green onions

Instructions:
1. Heat the sesame oil in a large pot over medium heat.
2. Add the chopped onion and cook until translucent, about 5 minutes.
3. Add the garlic and grated ginger, cooking for another minute until fragrant.
4. Stir in the cubed tofu, chopped bok choy, sliced carrots, and sliced mushrooms.
5. Pour in the vegetable broth, soy sauce, and rice vinegar. Bring to a boil.
6. Reduce heat and simmer for 20-25 minutes until the vegetables are tender.
7. If using, dissolve the miso paste in a small amount of hot broth, then stir it into the stew.
8. Stir in the chopped green onions before serving.
9. Serve hot.

Nutrition Info (per serving):
- Calories: 210
- Protein: 10g
- Carbohydrates: 18g
- Fiber: 4g
- Sugars: 6g
- Fat: 12g
- Saturated Fat: 2g

Serves: 4
Cooking Time: 35 minutes

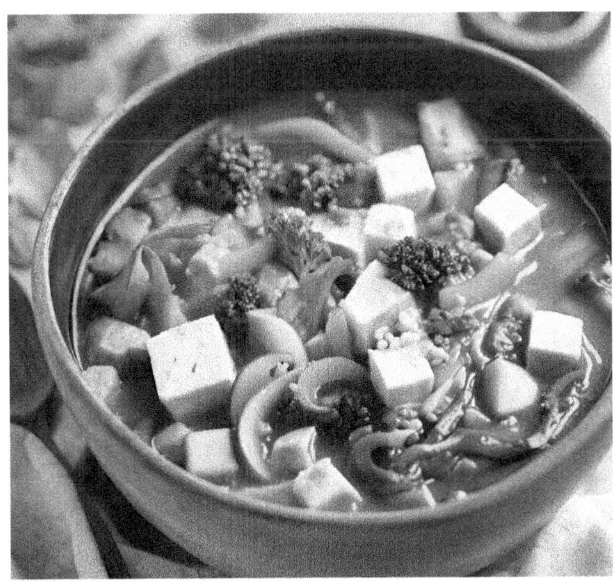

10. Sorrel Soup

Ingredients:

- 2 tablespoons olive oil
- 1 large onion, chopped
- 3 cloves garlic, minced
- 4 cups fresh sorrel leaves, chopped
- 4 cups low-sodium vegetable broth
- 2 cups diced potatoes
- 1 teaspoon dried thyme
- 1/4 cup unsweetened almond milk
- 1 tablespoon lemon juice

Instructions:

1. Heat the olive oil in a large pot over medium heat.
2. Add the chopped onion and cook until translucent, about 5 minutes.
3. Add the garlic and cook for another minute until fragrant.
4. Stir in the chopped sorrel leaves and cook until wilted, about 3-4 minutes.
5. Add the vegetable broth, diced potatoes, and thyme. Bring to a boil.
6. Reduce heat and simmer for 20-25 minutes until the potatoes are tender.
7. Use an immersion blender to puree the soup until smooth, or carefully transfer to a blender in batches and blend until smooth.
8. Stir in the almond milk and lemon juice.
9. Serve hot.

Nutrition Info (per serving):

- Calories: 170
- Protein: 4g
- Carbohydrates: 24g
- Fiber: 4g
- Sugars: 4g
- Fat: 7g
- Saturated Fat: 1g

Serves: 4

Cooking Time: 35 minutes

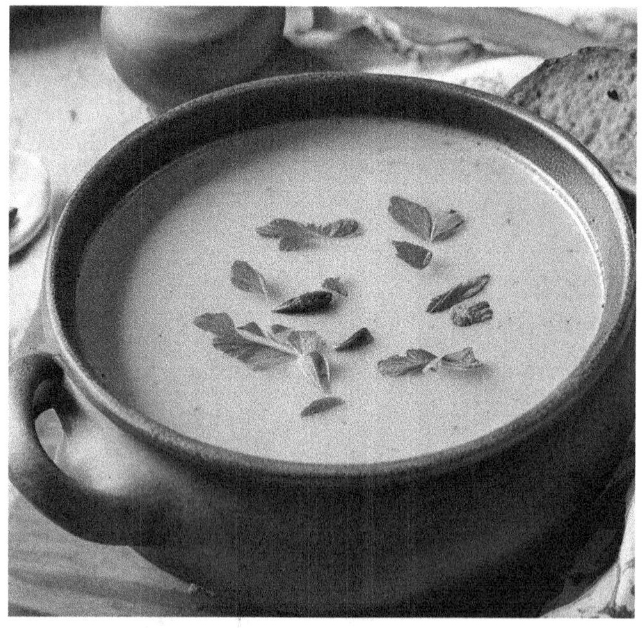

Poultry Recipes

1. Herb-Roasted Chicken Breast

Ingredients:

- 4 boneless, skinless chicken breasts
- 2 tablespoons olive oil
- 2 tablespoons chopped fresh rosemary
- 2 tablespoons chopped fresh thyme
- 2 cloves garlic, minced
- 1 tablespoon lemon juice
- 1 teaspoon paprika

Instructions:

1. Preheat the oven to 375°F (190°C).
2. In a small bowl, mix the olive oil, chopped rosemary, chopped thyme, minced garlic, lemon juice, and paprika.
3. Rub the mixture evenly over the chicken breasts.
4. Place the chicken breasts in a baking dish.
5. Bake in the preheated oven for 25-30 minutes, until the chicken is cooked through and the internal temperature reaches 165°F (74°C).
6. Let the chicken rest for 5 minutes before serving.

Nutrition Info (per serving):

- Calories: 220
- Protein: 26g
- Carbohydrates: 1g
- Fiber: 0g
- Sugars: 0g
- Fat: 12g
- Saturated Fat: 2g

Serves: 4
Cooking Time: 35 minutes

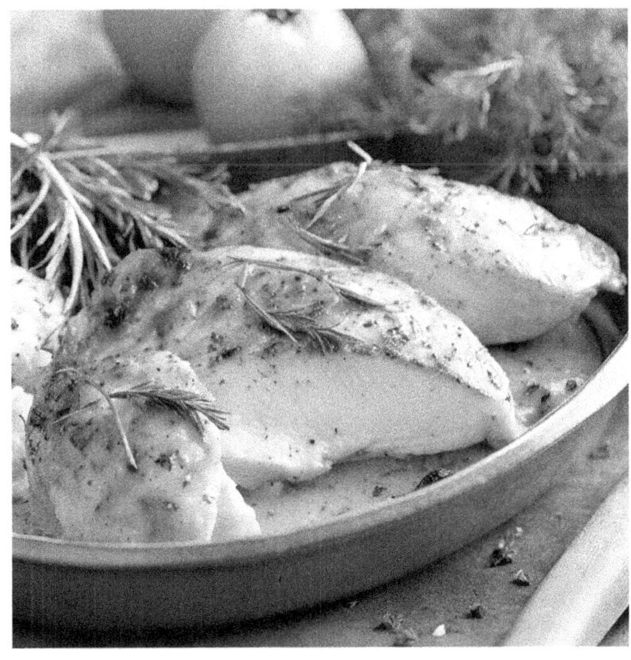

2. Chicken and Vegetable Stir-Fry

Ingredients:

- 2 tablespoons sesame oil
- 1 pound boneless, skinless chicken breasts, thinly sliced
- 1 large onion, sliced
- 2 cloves garlic, minced
- 1 tablespoon grated ginger
- 1 red bell pepper, sliced
- 1 yellow bell pepper, sliced
- 1 cup broccoli florets
- 1 cup snap peas
- 2 tablespoons low-sodium soy sauce
- 1 tablespoon rice vinegar
- 1 tablespoon honey

Instructions:

1. Heat 1 tablespoon of sesame oil in a large skillet or wok over medium-high heat.
2. Add the sliced chicken and cook until no longer pink, about 5-7 minutes. Remove the chicken from the skillet and set aside.
3. Add the remaining sesame oil to the skillet. Add the sliced onion, garlic, and grated ginger, cooking for 2-3 minutes until fragrant.
4. Add the red bell pepper, yellow bell pepper, broccoli florets, and snap peas. Stir-fry for 5-7 minutes until the vegetables are tender-crisp.
5. Return the chicken to the skillet.
6. In a small bowl, mix the soy sauce, rice vinegar, and honey. Pour the sauce over the chicken and vegetables, stirring to coat evenly.
7. Cook for another 2-3 minutes until everything is heated through.
8. Serve immediately.

Nutrition Info (per serving):

- Calories: 280
- Protein: 28g
- Carbohydrates: 18g
- Fiber: 4g
- Sugars: 10g
- Fat: 11g
- Saturated Fat: 2g

Serves: 4

Cooking Time: 25 minutes

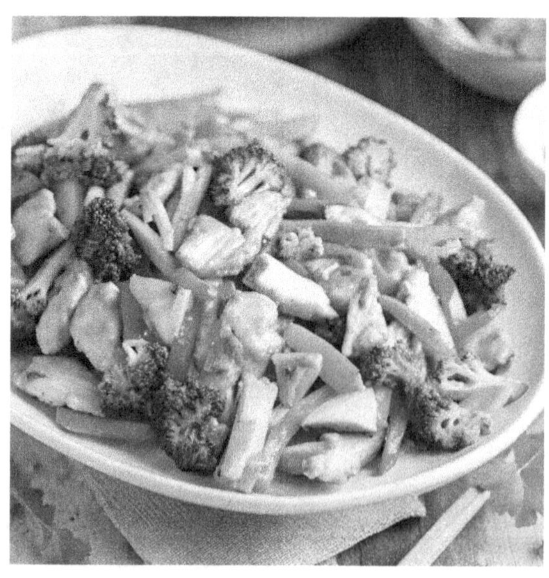

3. Lemon Garlic Chicken

Ingredients:

- 4 boneless, skinless chicken breasts
- 2 tablespoons olive oil
- 3 cloves garlic, minced
- Juice of 2 lemons
- 1 tablespoon lemon zest
- 1 tablespoon chopped fresh parsley
- 1 teaspoon dried oregano

Instructions:

1. Preheat the oven to 375°F (190°C).
2. In a small bowl, mix the olive oil, minced garlic, lemon juice, lemon zest, chopped parsley, and dried oregano.
3. Place the chicken breasts in a baking dish and pour the lemon garlic mixture over them.
4. Bake in the preheated oven for 25-30 minutes, until the chicken is cooked through and the internal temperature reaches 165°F (74°C).
5. Let the chicken rest for 5 minutes before serving.

Nutrition Info (per serving):

- Calories: 210
- Protein: 26g
- Carbohydrates: 2g
- Fiber: 0g
- Sugars: 0g
- Fat: 11g
- Saturated Fat: 2g

Serves: 4
Cooking Time: 35 minutes

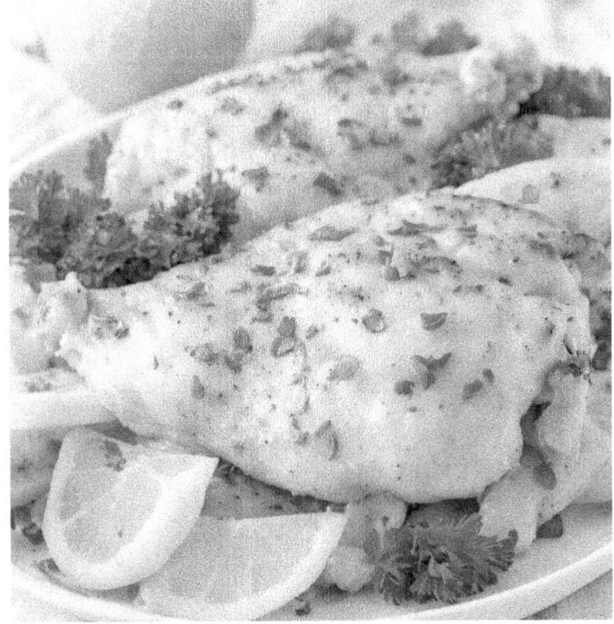

4. Chicken Soup with Vegetables

Ingredients:

- 2 tablespoons olive oil
- 1 pound boneless, skinless chicken breasts, diced
- 1 large onion, chopped
- 3 cloves garlic, minced
- 3 carrots, sliced
- 3 celery stalks, sliced
- 1 cup chopped tomatoes
- 6 cups low-sodium chicken broth
- 1 teaspoon dried thyme
- 1 teaspoon dried oregano
- 2 cups chopped spinach

Instructions:

1. Heat the olive oil in a large pot over medium heat.
2. Add the diced chicken and cook until no longer pink, about 5-7 minutes. Remove the chicken from the pot and set aside.
3. Add the chopped onion, garlic, carrots, and celery to the pot. Cook for 5-7 minutes until the vegetables are tender.
4. Stir in the chopped tomatoes, chicken broth, thyme, and oregano. Bring to a boil.
5. Reduce heat and simmer for 20 minutes.
6. Return the cooked chicken to the pot and add the chopped spinach. Cook for an additional 5 minutes until the spinach is wilted.
7. Serve hot.

Nutrition Info (per serving):

- Calories: 200
- Protein: 24g
- Carbohydrates: 12g
- Fiber: 3g
- Sugars: 5g
- Fat: 7g
- Saturated Fat: 1.5g

Serves: 6

Cooking Time: 40 minutes

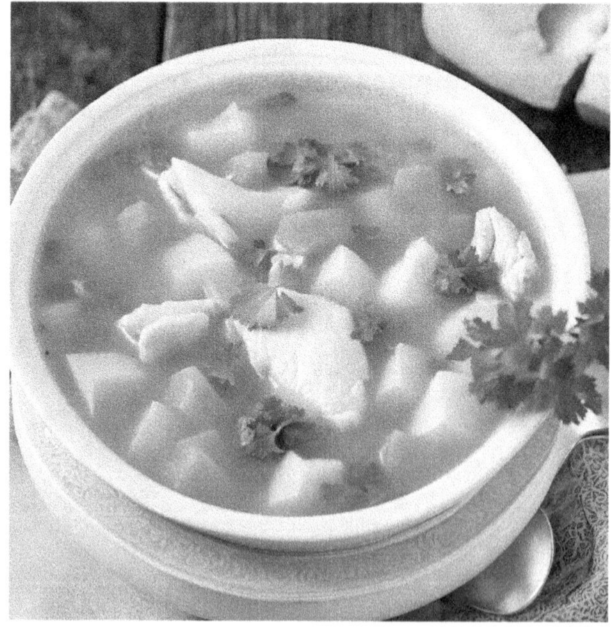

5. Grilled Chicken Salad

Ingredients:

- 2 boneless, skinless chicken breasts
- 2 tablespoons olive oil
- 1 tablespoon lemon juice
- 1 teaspoon dried oregano
- 4 cups mixed salad greens
- 1 cup cherry tomatoes, halved
- 1 cucumber, sliced
- 1/4 cup red onion, thinly sliced
- 1/4 cup feta cheese, crumbled
- 2 tablespoons balsamic vinegar

Instructions:

1. Preheat the grill to medium-high heat.
2. In a small bowl, mix 1 tablespoon of olive oil, lemon juice, and dried oregano. Brush the mixture over the chicken breasts.
3. Grill the chicken breasts for 6-7 minutes on each side, until cooked through and the internal temperature reaches 165°F (74°C). Let rest for 5 minutes, then slice.
4. In a large bowl, combine the mixed salad greens, cherry tomatoes, cucumber, red onion, and feta cheese.
5. Add the grilled chicken slices on top.
6. Drizzle with the remaining olive oil and balsamic vinegar.
7. Toss gently and serve immediately.

Nutrition Info (per serving):

- Calories: 300
- Protein: 25g
- Carbohydrates: 10g
- Fiber: 3g
- Sugars: 4g
- Fat: 18g
- Saturated Fat: 4g

Serves: 2
Cooking Time: 20 minutes

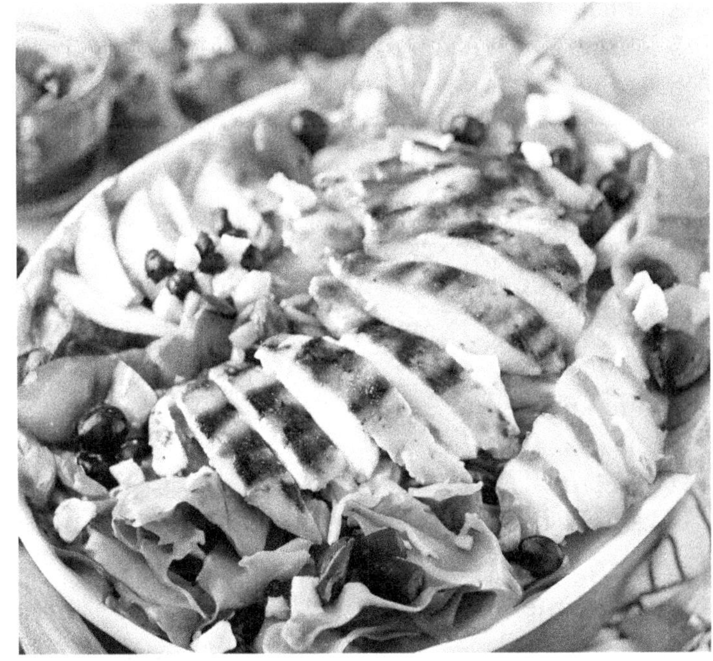

6. Moroccan Chicken Tagine

Ingredients:

- 2 tablespoons olive oil
- 1 pound boneless, skinless chicken thighs, cut into chunks
- 1 large onion, chopped
- 3 cloves garlic, minced
- 2 carrots, sliced
- 1 red bell pepper, chopped
- 1 cup chopped tomatoes
- 1 cup low-sodium chicken broth
- 1/4 cup dried apricots, chopped
- 1 teaspoon ground cumin
- 1 teaspoon ground coriander
- 1/2 teaspoon ground cinnamon
- 1/2 teaspoon ground turmeric
- 1/4 cup chopped fresh cilantro

Instructions:

1. Heat the olive oil in a large pot or tagine over medium heat.
2. Add the chicken thighs and cook until browned on all sides, about 5-7 minutes. Remove from the pot and set aside.
3. Add the chopped onion, garlic, carrots, and red bell pepper to the pot. Cook for 5-7 minutes until the vegetables are tender.
4. Stir in the chopped tomatoes, chicken broth, dried apricots, cumin, coriander, cinnamon, and turmeric.
5. Return the chicken to the pot and bring to a boil.
6. Reduce heat, cover, and simmer for 30-35 minutes, until the chicken is cooked through and tender.
7. Stir in the chopped fresh cilantro before serving.
8. Serve hot.

Nutrition Info (per serving):

- Calories: 320
- Protein: 25g
- Carbohydrates: 25g
- Fiber: 6g
- Sugars: 12g
- Fat: 14g
- Saturated Fat: 2.5g

Serves: 4
Cooking Time: 45 minutes

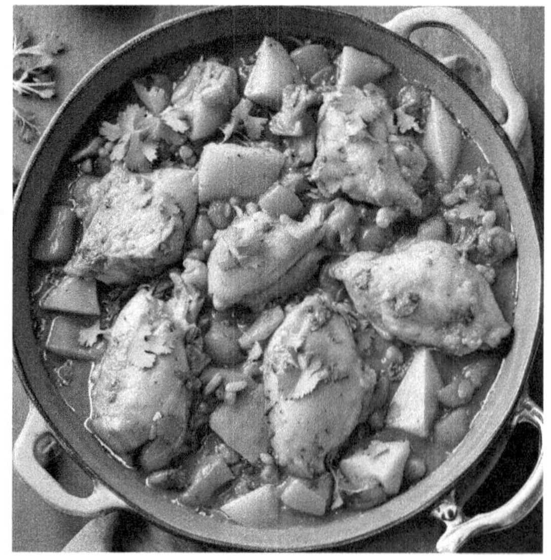

7. Baked Chicken with Brussels Sprouts

Ingredients:

- 4 boneless, skinless chicken breasts
- 2 tablespoons olive oil
- 1 pound Brussels sprouts, trimmed and halved
- 1 large onion, chopped
- 3 cloves garlic, minced
- 1 teaspoon dried thyme
- 1 tablespoon lemon juice

Instructions:

1. Preheat the oven to 400°F (200°C).
2. In a large bowl, toss the Brussels sprouts, chopped onion, and minced garlic with 1 tablespoon of olive oil and dried thyme.
3. Spread the vegetable mixture evenly on a baking sheet.
4. Rub the chicken breasts with the remaining olive oil and place them on top of the vegetable mixture.
5. Bake in the preheated oven for 25-30 minutes, until the chicken is cooked through and the internal temperature reaches 165°F (74°C).
6. Drizzle with lemon juice before serving.
7. Serve hot.

Nutrition Info (per serving):

- Calories: 280
- Protein: 29g
- Carbohydrates: 14g
- Fiber: 5g
- Sugars: 4g
- Fat: 12g
- Saturated Fat: 2g

Serves: 4
Cooking Time: 35 minutes

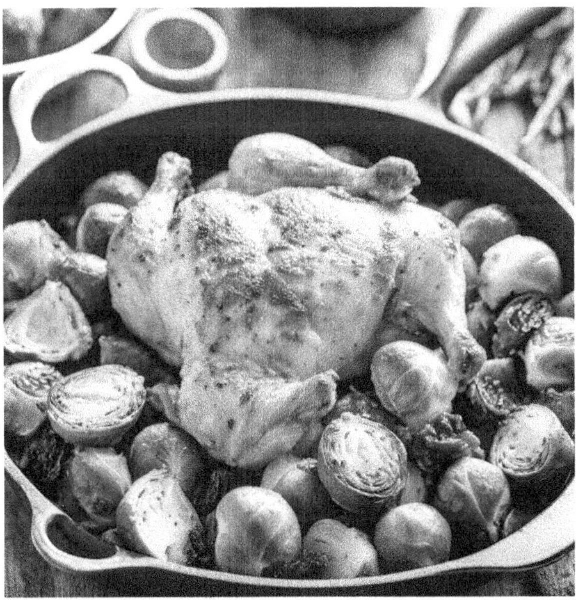

8. Turkey Chili

Ingredients:

- 2 tablespoons olive oil
- 1 pound ground turkey
- 1 large onion, chopped
- 3 cloves garlic, minced
- 1 red bell pepper, chopped
- 1 green bell pepper, chopped
- 1 can (15 oz) black beans, rinsed and drained
- 1 can (15 oz) kidney beans, rinsed and drained
- 2 cups chopped tomatoes
- 2 cups low-sodium chicken broth
- 1 tablespoon chili powder
- 1 teaspoon ground cumin
- 1 teaspoon smoked paprika
- 1/2 teaspoon ground oregano
- 1/4 cup chopped fresh cilantro

Instructions:

1. Heat the olive oil in a large pot over medium heat.
2. Add the ground turkey and cook until browned, about 5-7 minutes.
3. Add the chopped onion, garlic, red bell pepper, and green bell pepper. Cook for 5-7 minutes until the vegetables are tender.
4. Stir in the black beans, kidney beans, chopped tomatoes, chicken broth, chili powder, cumin, smoked paprika, and oregano.
5. Bring to a boil, then reduce heat and simmer for 30-35 minutes, until the chili is thickened.
6. Stir in the chopped fresh cilantro before serving.
7. Serve hot.

Nutrition Info (per serving):

- Calories: 320
- Protein: 26g
- Carbohydrates: 28g
- Fiber: 10g
- Sugars: 7g
- Fat: 12g
- Saturated Fat: 2.5g

Serves: 4

Cooking Time: 45 minutes

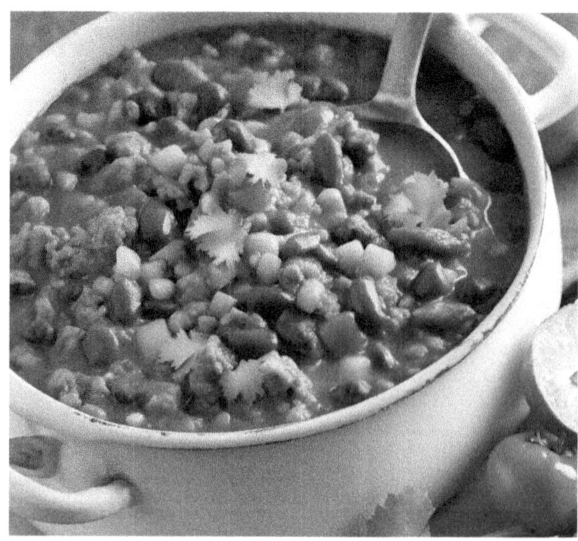

9. Turkey Meatballs

Ingredients:

- 1 pound ground turkey
- 1/4 cup whole grain breadcrumbs
- 1/4 cup grated Parmesan cheese
- 1 egg, lightly beaten
- 2 cloves garlic, minced
- 1 teaspoon dried oregano
- 1 tablespoon chopped fresh parsley
- 2 tablespoons olive oil
- 2 cups marinara sauce (low sodium)

Instructions:

1. Preheat the oven to 375°F (190°C).
2. In a large bowl, combine the ground turkey, breadcrumbs, Parmesan cheese, beaten egg, minced garlic, dried oregano, and chopped parsley. Mix well.
3. Form the mixture into 12 meatballs.
4. Heat the olive oil in a large skillet over medium heat.
5. Add the meatballs and cook until browned on all sides, about 5-7 minutes.
6. Transfer the meatballs to a baking dish and pour the marinara sauce over them.
7. Bake in the preheated oven for 20-25 minutes, until the meatballs are cooked through and the internal temperature reaches 165°F (74°C).
8. Serve hot.

Nutrition Info (per serving):

- Calories: 250
- Protein: 22g
- Carbohydrates: 12g
- Fiber: 2g
- Sugars: 5g
- Fat: 12g
- Saturated Fat: 3g

Serves: 4
Cooking Time: 35 minutes

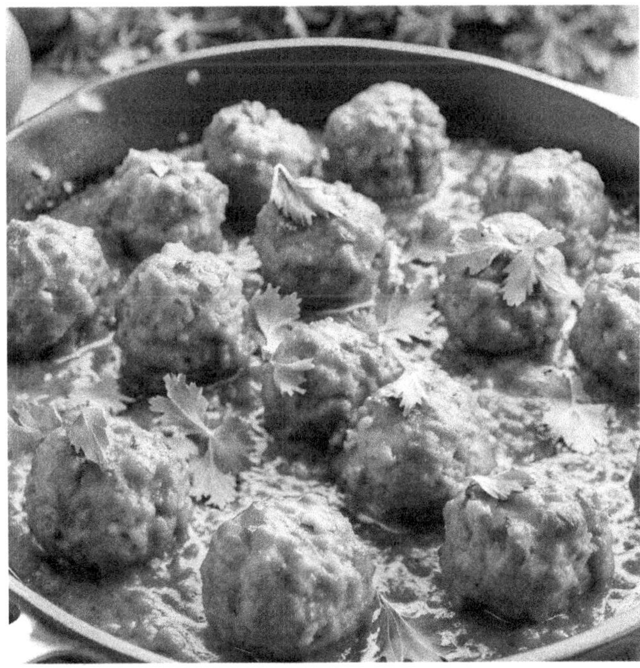

10. Stuffed Turkey Breast

Ingredients:

- 1 boneless turkey breast (about 2 pounds)
- 2 tablespoons olive oil
- 1 cup cooked quinoa
- 1/2 cup dried cranberries (unsweetened)
- 1/4 cup chopped walnuts
- 1/4 cup chopped fresh parsley
- 1 teaspoon dried thyme
- 1 teaspoon dried sage
- 1/2 cup low-sodium chicken broth

Instructions:

1. Preheat the oven to 375°F (190°C).
2. Butterfly the turkey breast and pound it to an even thickness.
3. In a bowl, mix the cooked quinoa, dried cranberries, chopped walnuts, fresh parsley, dried thyme, and dried sage.
4. Spread the quinoa mixture over the turkey breast, then roll it up and secure with kitchen twine.
5. Heat the olive oil in an oven-safe skillet over medium-high heat. Brown the turkey breast on all sides, about 5-7 minutes.
6. Add the chicken broth to the skillet, then transfer it to the preheated oven.
7. Bake for 25-30 minutes, until the internal temperature reaches 165°F (74°C).
8. Let the turkey rest for 10 minutes before slicing and serving.

Nutrition Info (per serving):

- Calories: 280
- Protein: 28g
- Carbohydrates: 16g
- Fiber: 3g
- Sugars: 7g
- Fat: 12g
- Saturated Fat: 2g

Serves: 4

Cooking Time: 45 minutes

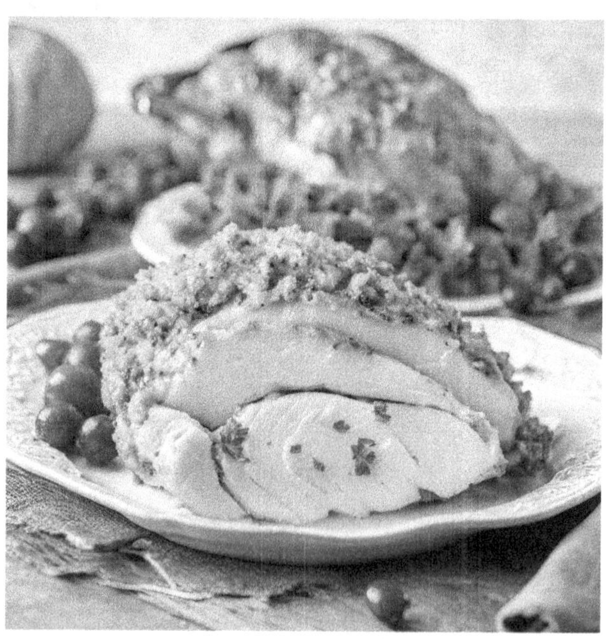

11. Turkey and Sweet Potato Skillet

Ingredients:

- 2 tablespoons olive oil
- 1 pound ground turkey
- 1 large onion, chopped
- 2 cloves garlic, minced
- 2 medium sweet potatoes, peeled and diced
- 1 red bell pepper, chopped
- 1 teaspoon ground cumin
- 1/2 teaspoon paprika
- 1/4 cup chopped fresh cilantro
- 1 tablespoon lime juice

Instructions:

1. Heat the olive oil in a large skillet over medium heat.
2. Add the ground turkey and cook until browned, about 5-7 minutes.
3. Add the chopped onion and minced garlic, cooking for another 3-4 minutes until softened.
4. Stir in the diced sweet potatoes, red bell pepper, ground cumin, and paprika.
5. Cover and cook for 15-20 minutes, stirring occasionally, until the sweet potatoes are tender.
6. Stir in the chopped fresh cilantro and lime juice before serving.
7. Serve hot.

Nutrition Info (per serving):

- Calories: 320
- Protein: 25g
- Carbohydrates: 30g
- Fiber: 5g
- Sugars: 8g
- Fat: 12g
- Saturated Fat: 2g

Serves: 4
Cooking Time: 30 minutes

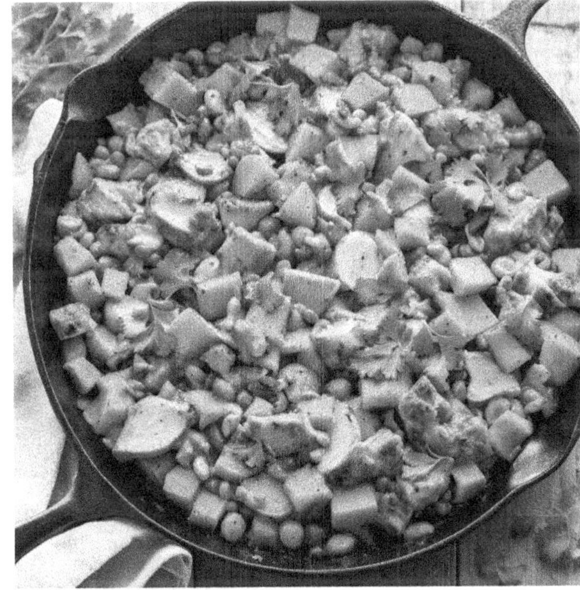

12. Smoked Turkey and Bean Soup

Ingredients:

- 2 tablespoons olive oil
- 1 large onion, chopped
- 2 cloves garlic, minced
- 2 carrots, sliced
- 2 celery stalks, sliced
- 1 smoked turkey leg, skin removed and meat shredded
- 2 cans (15 oz each) white beans, rinsed and drained
- 4 cups low-sodium chicken broth
- 1 teaspoon dried thyme
- 1 teaspoon smoked paprika
- 1/4 cup chopped fresh parsley

Instructions:

1. Heat the olive oil in a large pot over medium heat.
2. Add the chopped onion and cook until translucent, about 5 minutes.
3. Add the minced garlic, sliced carrots, and sliced celery, cooking for another 5 minutes until softened.
4. Stir in the shredded smoked turkey, white beans, chicken broth, dried thyme, and smoked paprika.
5. Bring to a boil, then reduce heat and simmer for 25-30 minutes.
6. Stir in the chopped fresh parsley before serving.
7. Serve hot.

Nutrition Info (per serving):

- Calories: 280
- Protein: 25g
- Carbohydrates: 24g
- Fiber: 8g
- Sugars: 4g
- Fat: 10g
- Saturated Fat: 2g

Serves: 6

Cooking Time: 45 minutes

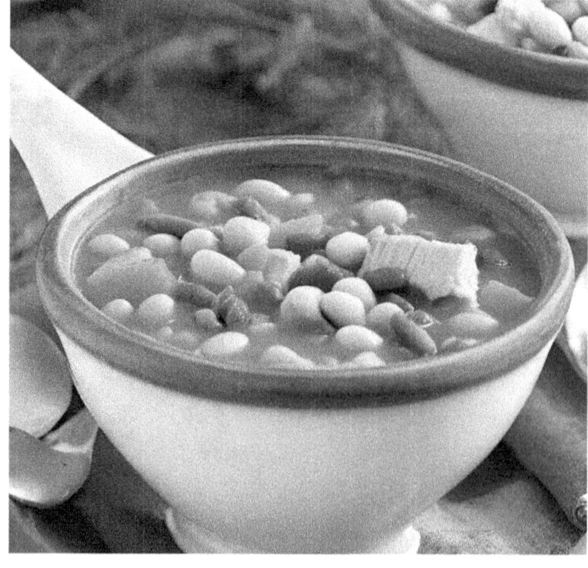

13. Turkey and Quinoa Stuffed Peppers

Ingredients:

- 4 large bell peppers
- 2 tablespoons olive oil
- 1 pound ground turkey
- 1 large onion, chopped
- 2 cloves garlic, minced
- 1 cup cooked quinoa
- 1 can (15 oz) diced tomatoes, no salt added
- 1 teaspoon ground cumin
- 1 teaspoon dried oregano
- 1/4 cup chopped fresh parsley

Instructions:

1. Preheat the oven to 375°F (190°C).
2. Cut the tops off the bell peppers and remove the seeds. Place them in a baking dish.
3. Heat the olive oil in a large skillet over medium heat. Add the ground turkey and cook until browned, about 5-7 minutes.
4. Add the chopped onion and minced garlic, cooking for another 3-4 minutes until softened.
5. Stir in the cooked quinoa, diced tomatoes, ground cumin, and dried oregano. Cook for another 5 minutes.
6. Spoon the turkey mixture into the bell peppers.
7. Cover with foil and bake in the preheated oven for 30 minutes. Remove the foil and bake for an additional 10 minutes.
8. Sprinkle with chopped fresh parsley before serving.
9. Serve hot.

Nutrition Info (per serving):

- Calories: 300
- Protein: 25g
- Carbohydrates: 28g
- Fiber: 7g
- Sugars: 10g
- Fat: 12g
- Saturated Fat: 2g

Serves: 4
Cooking Time: 45 minutes

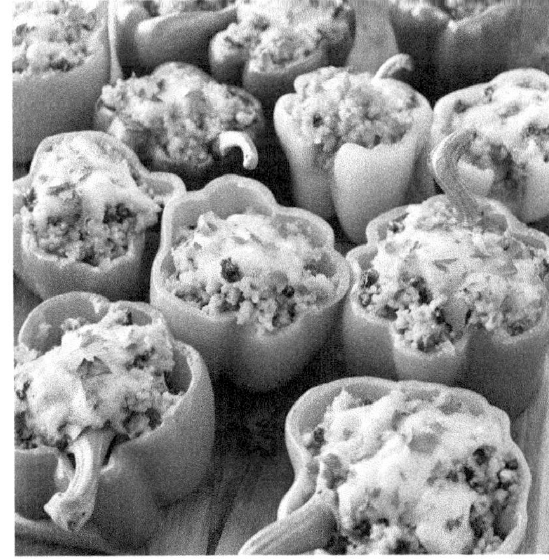

14. Turkish Turkey Kebabs

Ingredients:

- 1 pound ground turkey
- 1 small onion, grated
- 2 cloves garlic, minced
- 1 tablespoon chopped fresh mint
- 1 tablespoon chopped fresh parsley
- 1 teaspoon ground cumin
- 1/2 teaspoon ground coriander
- 1/2 teaspoon paprika
- 2 tablespoons olive oil

Instructions:

1. In a large bowl, combine the ground turkey, grated onion, minced garlic, chopped mint, chopped parsley, ground cumin, ground coriander, and paprika. Mix well.
2. Shape the mixture into 8-10 kebabs.
3. Preheat the grill to medium-high heat and brush with olive oil.
4. Grill the kebabs for 6-8 minutes on each side, until cooked through and the internal temperature reaches 165°F (74°C).
5. Serve hot with a side of grilled vegetables or salad.

Nutrition Info (per serving):

- Calories: 200
- Protein: 22g
- Carbohydrates: 3g
- Fiber: 1g
- Sugars: 1g
- Fat: 12g
- Saturated Fat: 2.5g

Serves: 4
Cooking Time: 20 minutes

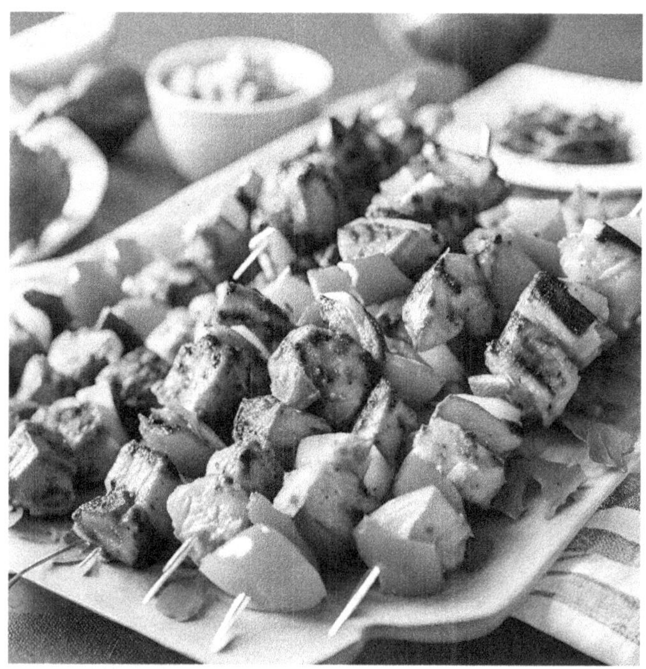

15. Turkey Vegetable Stir-Fry

Ingredients:

- 2 tablespoons sesame oil
- 1 pound ground turkey
- 1 large onion, chopped
- 2 cloves garlic, minced
- 1 red bell pepper, sliced
- 1 green bell pepper, sliced
- 1 cup broccoli florets
- 1 cup snap peas
- 2 tablespoons low-sodium soy sauce
- 1 tablespoon rice vinegar
- 1 tablespoon honey

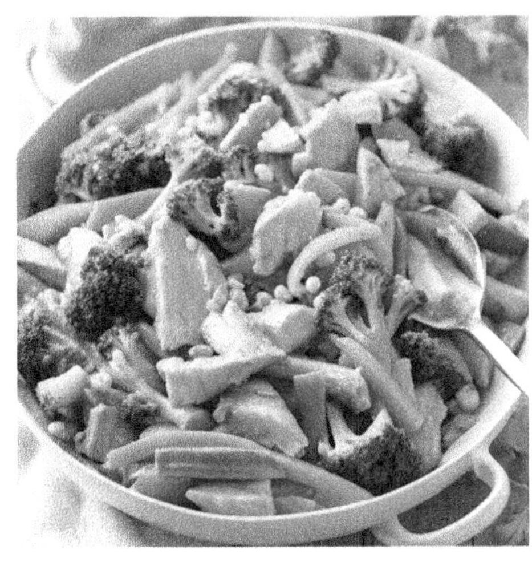

Instructions:

1. Heat 1 tablespoon of sesame oil in a large skillet or wok over medium-high heat.
2. Add the ground turkey and cook until browned, about 5-7 minutes. Remove the turkey from the skillet and set aside.
3. Add the remaining sesame oil to the skillet. Add the chopped onion, garlic, red bell pepper, and green bell pepper. Stir-fry for 5-7 minutes until the vegetables are tender-crisp.
4. Add the broccoli florets and snap peas, cooking for another 3-4 minutes.
5. Return the turkey to the skillet.
6. In a small bowl, mix the soy sauce, rice vinegar, and honey. Pour the sauce over the turkey and vegetables, stirring to coat evenly.
7. Cook for another 2-3 minutes until everything is heated through.
8. Serve immediately.

Nutrition Info (per serving):

- Calories: 280
- Protein: 25g
- Carbohydrates: 18g
- Fiber: 4g
- Sugars: 9g
- Fat: 12g
- Saturated Fat: 2g

Serves: 4
Cooking Time: 25 minutes

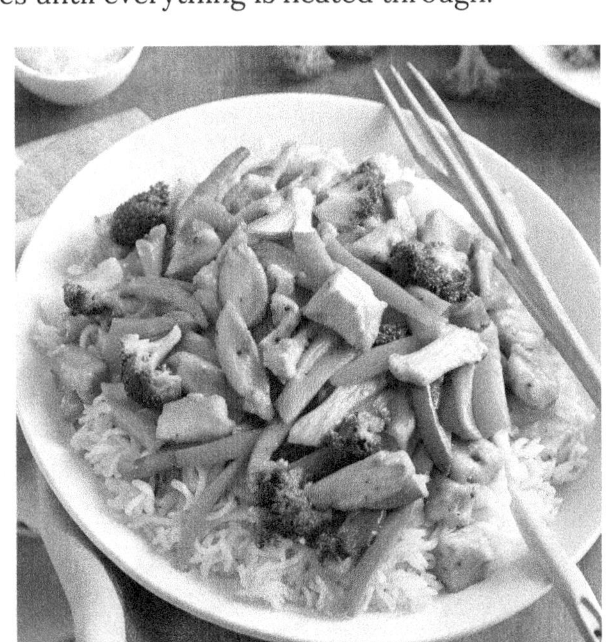

16. Duck Breast with Orange Sauce

Ingredients:

- 2 duck breasts
- 1/2 cup orange juice (freshly squeezed)
- 1 tablespoon honey
- 1 teaspoon Dijon mustard
- 1 tablespoon apple cider vinegar
- 1 tablespoon olive oil
- 1 teaspoon dried thyme
- 1 orange, thinly sliced

Instructions:

1. Preheat the oven to 375°F (190°C).
2. Score the skin of the duck breasts in a crisscross pattern, being careful not to cut into the meat.
3. Heat a skillet over medium-high heat and place the duck breasts skin side down. Cook for 5-7 minutes until the skin is crispy.
4. Flip the duck breasts and cook for an additional 3-4 minutes.
5. Transfer the duck breasts to a baking dish and bake in the preheated oven for 10-15 minutes until the internal temperature reaches 135°F (57°C) for medium-rare.
6. In the same skillet, add the orange juice, honey, Dijon mustard, and apple cider vinegar. Bring to a simmer and cook for 5 minutes until the sauce thickens.
7. Slice the duck breasts and serve with the orange sauce and orange slices.

Nutrition Info (per serving):

- Calories: 300
- Protein: 24g
- Carbohydrates: 12g
- Fiber: 1g
- Sugars: 10g
- Fat: 18g
- Saturated Fat: 5g

Serves: 2

Cooking Time: 30 minutes

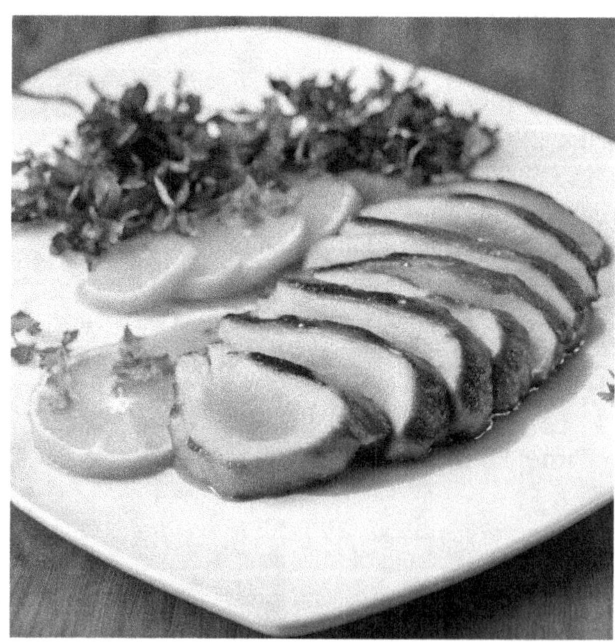

17. Balsamic Glazed Chicken Thighs
Ingredients:
- 4 boneless, skinless chicken thighs
- 2 tablespoons olive oil
- 1/4 cup balsamic vinegar
- 2 tablespoons honey
- 1 teaspoon dried rosemary
- 3 cloves garlic, minced

Instructions:
1. Preheat the oven to 375°F (190°C).
2. In a small bowl, mix the balsamic vinegar, honey, dried rosemary, and minced garlic.
3. Heat the olive oil in an oven-safe skillet over medium-high heat. Add the chicken thighs and cook for 5-7 minutes on each side until browned.
4. Pour the balsamic mixture over the chicken thighs.
5. Transfer the skillet to the preheated oven and bake for 20-25 minutes until the chicken is cooked through and the internal temperature reaches 165°F (74°C).
6. Serve hot with the glaze spooned over the chicken.

Nutrition Info (per serving):
- Calories: 250
- Protein: 20g
- Carbohydrates: 12g
- Fiber: 0g
- Sugars: 10g
- Fat: 14g
- Saturated Fat: 3g

Serves: 4
Cooking Time: 35 minutes

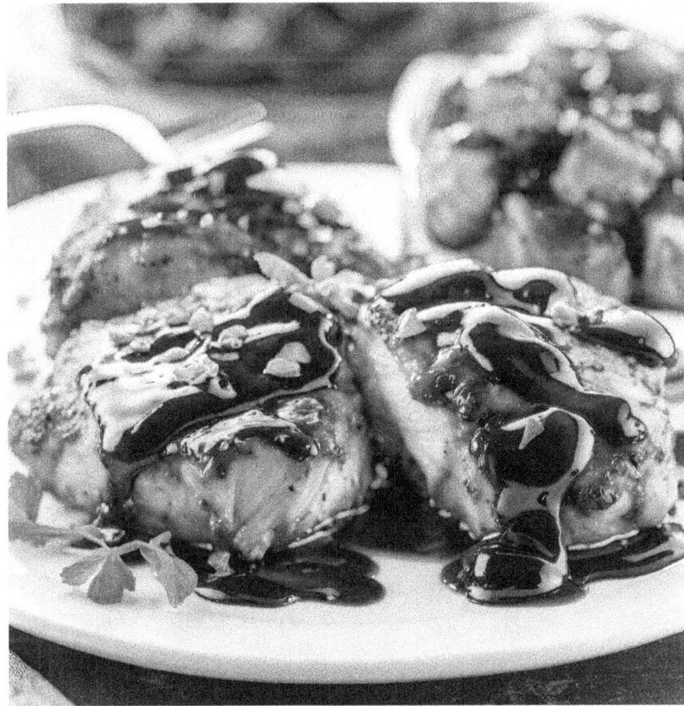

18. Chicken Paillard

Ingredients:

- 4 boneless, skinless chicken breasts
- 2 tablespoons olive oil
- 1 tablespoon lemon juice
- 1 teaspoon dried oregano
- 2 cloves garlic, minced
- 4 cups mixed salad greens
- 1 cup cherry tomatoes, halved
- 1/4 cup red onion, thinly sliced

Instructions:

1. Place the chicken breasts between two pieces of plastic wrap and pound them to an even thickness.
2. In a small bowl, mix the olive oil, lemon juice, dried oregano, and minced garlic.
3. Brush the mixture over the chicken breasts.
4. Heat a large skillet over medium-high heat. Add the chicken breasts and cook for 4-5 minutes on each side until cooked through and the internal temperature reaches 165°F (74°C).
5. In a large bowl, toss the salad greens, cherry tomatoes, and red onion.
6. Serve the chicken paillard on top of the salad.

Nutrition Info (per serving):

- Calories: 220
- Protein: 25g
- Carbohydrates: 6g
- Fiber: 2g
- Sugars: 2g
- Fat: 12g
- Saturated Fat: 2g

Serves: 4

Cooking Time: 20 minutes

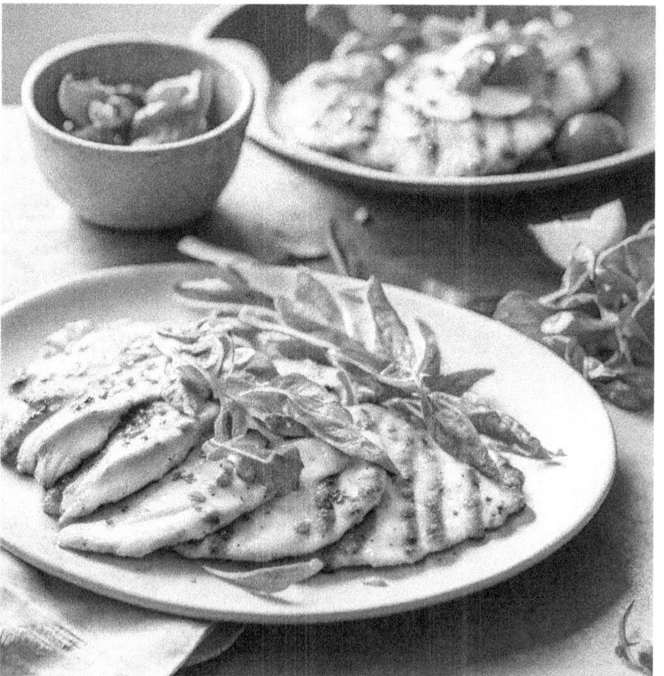

19. Chicken Fajitas

Ingredients:

- 1 pound boneless, skinless chicken breasts, thinly sliced
- 2 tablespoons olive oil
- 1 teaspoon ground cumin
- 1 teaspoon paprika
- 1 teaspoon dried oregano
- 1 red bell pepper, sliced
- 1 yellow bell pepper, sliced
- 1 large onion, sliced
- 8 whole grain tortillas
- 1 lime, cut into wedges
- 1/4 cup chopped fresh cilantro

Instructions:

1. In a large bowl, mix the olive oil, ground cumin, paprika, and dried oregano.
2. Add the sliced chicken breasts and toss to coat evenly.
3. Heat a large skillet over medium-high heat. Add the chicken and cook for 5-7 minutes until cooked through.
4. Remove the chicken from the skillet and set aside.
5. Add the sliced bell peppers and onion to the skillet. Cook for 5-7 minutes until tender.
6. Return the chicken to the skillet and toss to combine with the vegetables.
7. Serve the chicken and vegetables in whole grain tortillas, garnished with lime wedges and chopped cilantro.

Nutrition Info (per serving):

- Calories: 300
- Protein: 25g
- Carbohydrates: 30g
- Fiber: 6g
- Sugars: 4g
- Fat: 10g
- Saturated Fat: 2g

Serves: 4
Cooking Time: 25 minutes

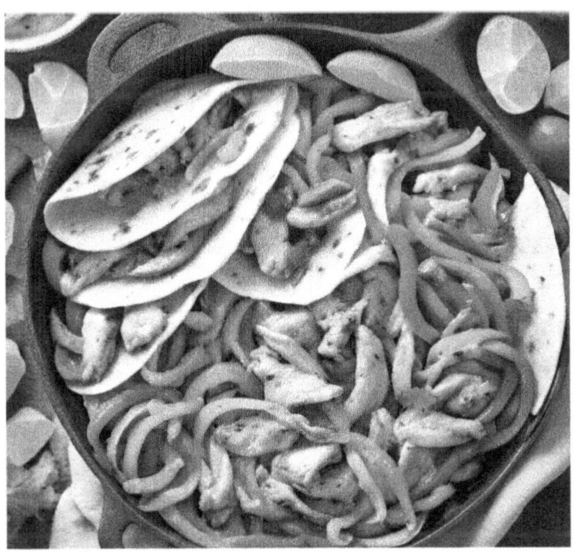

20. Chicken Cacciatore

Ingredients:

- 4 boneless, skinless chicken thighs
- 2 tablespoons olive oil
- 1 large onion, chopped
- 3 cloves garlic, minced
- 1 red bell pepper, chopped
- 1 yellow bell pepper, chopped
- 1 cup sliced mushrooms
- 1 cup chopped tomatoes
- 1 cup low-sodium chicken broth
- 1 teaspoon dried oregano
- 1 teaspoon dried thyme
- 1/4 cup chopped fresh parsley

Instructions:

1. Heat the olive oil in a large skillet over medium-high heat.
2. Add the chicken thighs and cook for 5-7 minutes on each side until browned. Remove from the skillet and set aside.
3. Add the chopped onion, garlic, bell peppers, and mushrooms to the skillet. Cook for 5-7 minutes until the vegetables are tender.
4. Stir in the chopped tomatoes, chicken broth, dried oregano, and dried thyme.
5. Return the chicken to the skillet and bring to a boil.
6. Reduce heat, cover, and simmer for 25-30 minutes until the chicken is cooked through and the sauce is thickened.
7. Stir in the chopped fresh parsley before serving.
8. Serve hot.

Nutrition Info (per serving):

- Calories: 280
- Protein: 25g
- Carbohydrates: 14g
- Fiber: 4g
- Sugars: 7g
- Fat: 14g
- Saturated Fat: 3g

Serves: 4
Cooking Time: 45 minutes

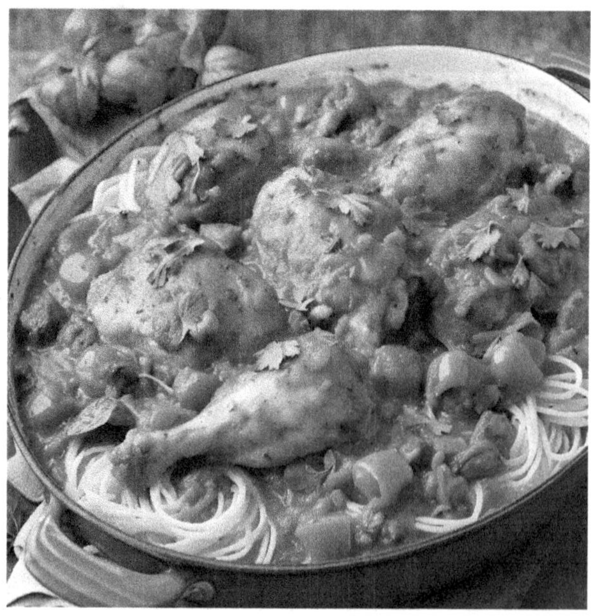

21. Chicken and Asparagus Lemon Stir Fry

Ingredients:

- 1 pound boneless, skinless chicken breasts, thinly sliced
- 2 tablespoons olive oil
- 2 cloves garlic, minced
- 1 bunch asparagus, trimmed and cut into 2-inch pieces
- 1 red bell pepper, sliced
- 2 tablespoons lemon juice
- 1 teaspoon lemon zest
- 1 teaspoon dried thyme
- 1 tablespoon low-sodium soy sauce

Instructions:

1. Heat 1 tablespoon of olive oil in a large skillet over medium-high heat.
2. Add the chicken slices and cook until browned and cooked through, about 5-7 minutes. Remove the chicken from the skillet and set aside.
3. Add the remaining olive oil to the skillet. Add the minced garlic, asparagus, and red bell pepper. Cook for 5-7 minutes until the vegetables are tender-crisp.
4. Return the chicken to the skillet. Stir in the lemon juice, lemon zest, thyme, and soy sauce.
5. Cook for an additional 2-3 minutes until everything is heated through.
6. Serve immediately.

Nutrition Info (per serving):

- Calories: 250
- Protein: 25g
- Carbohydratcs: 10g
- Fiber: 4g
- Sugars: 3g
- Fat: 12g
- Saturated Fat: 2g

Serves: 4
Cooking Time: 20 minutes

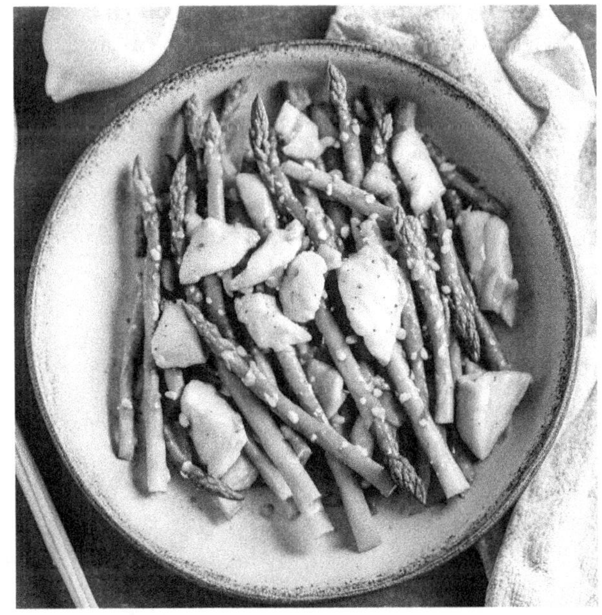

22. Buffalo Chicken Stuffed Zucchini

Ingredients:

- 4 medium zucchinis
- 1 pound ground chicken
- 2 tablespoons olive oil
- 1 large onion, chopped
- 2 cloves garlic, minced
- 1/2 cup hot sauce (such as Frank's RedHot)
- 1/4 cup low-fat Greek yogurt
- 1/4 cup crumbled blue cheese
- 1 tablespoon chopped fresh parsley

Instructions:

1. Preheat the oven to 375°F (190°C).
2. Cut the zucchinis in half lengthwise and scoop out the seeds to create boats.
3. In a large skillet, heat the olive oil over medium heat. Add the ground chicken, chopped onion, and minced garlic. Cook until the chicken is browned, about 5-7 minutes.
4. Stir in the hot sauce and Greek yogurt, cooking for another 2 minutes until well combined.
5. Stuff the zucchini halves with the chicken mixture and place them in a baking dish.
6. Sprinkle with crumbled blue cheese.
7. Bake in the preheated oven for 25-30 minutes until the zucchinis are tender.
8. Garnish with chopped fresh parsley before serving.
9. Serve hot.

Nutrition Info (per serving):

- Calories: 280
- Protein: 28g
- Carbohydrates: 10g
- Fiber: 2g
- Sugars: 5g
- Fat: 14g
- Saturated Fat: 4g

Serves: 4

Cooking Time: 40 minutes

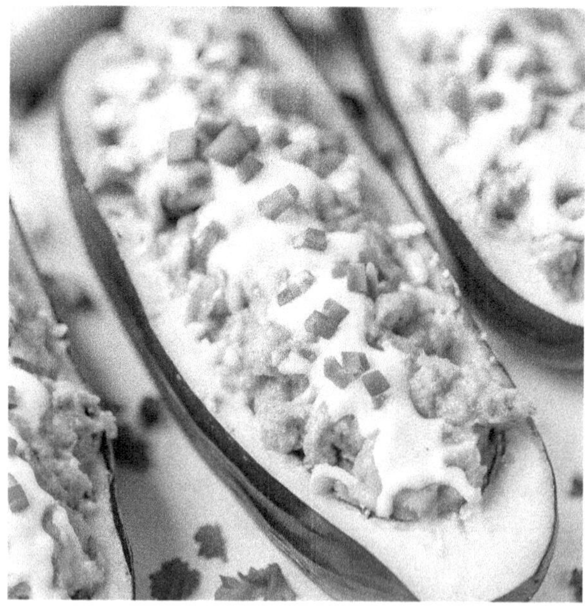

23. Chicken and Broccoli Alfredo

Ingredients:
- 1 pound boneless, skinless chicken breasts, thinly sliced
- 2 tablespoons olive oil
- 2 cloves garlic, minced
- 4 cups broccoli florets
- 1 cup low-fat milk
- 1/2 cup grated Parmesan cheese
- 1/4 cup low-fat Greek yogurt
- 1 teaspoon dried basil
- 8 ounces whole grain pasta

Instructions:
1. Cook the pasta according to package instructions. Drain and set aside.
2. Heat 1 tablespoon of olive oil in a large skillet over medium-high heat. Add the chicken slices and cook until browned and cooked through, about 5-7 minutes. Remove the chicken from the skillet and set aside.
3. Add the remaining olive oil to the skillet. Add the minced garlic and cook for 1 minute until fragrant.
4. Add the broccoli florets and cook for 5-7 minutes until tender.
5. Stir in the milk, Parmesan cheese, Greek yogurt, and dried basil. Cook for 3-4 minutes until the sauce thickens.
6. Return the chicken to the skillet and toss to coat in the sauce.
7. Serve the chicken and broccoli Alfredo over the cooked pasta.

Nutrition Info (per serving):
- Calorics: 400
- Protein: 32g
- Carbohydratcs: 45g
- Fiber: 8g
- Sugars: 6g
- Fat: 12g
- Saturated Fat: 3g

Serves: 4
Cooking Time: 30 minutes

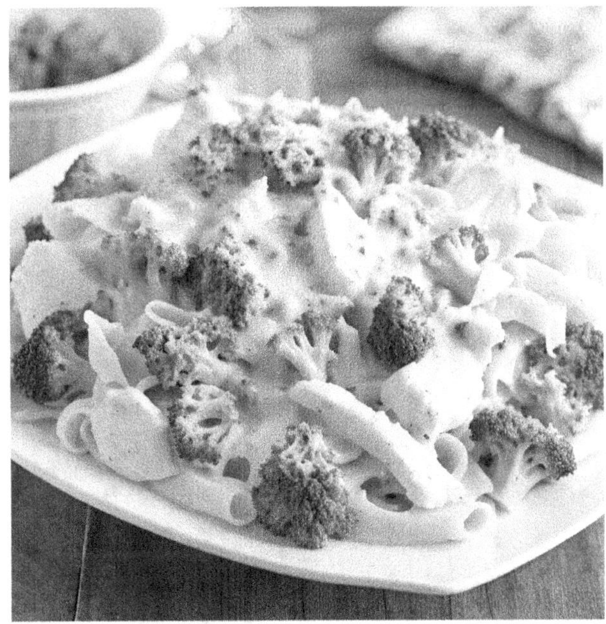

24. Mediterranean Turkey Meatloaf

Ingredients:

- 1 pound ground turkey
- 1/2 cup whole grain breadcrumbs
- 1/4 cup grated Parmesan cheese
- 1/4 cup chopped sun-dried tomatoes (not in oil)
- 1/4 cup chopped Kalamata olives
- 1/4 cup chopped fresh parsley
- 1 egg, lightly beaten
- 1 teaspoon dried oregano
- 1 teaspoon dried basil
- 1 tablespoon olive oil

Instructions:

1. Preheat the oven to 375°F (190°C).
2. In a large bowl, combine the ground turkey, breadcrumbs, Parmesan cheese, sun-dried tomatoes, Kalamata olives, chopped parsley, beaten egg, dried oregano, and dried basil. Mix well.
3. Form the mixture into a loaf and place it in a greased loaf pan.
4. Brush the top with olive oil.
5. Bake in the preheated oven for 45-50 minutes until the internal temperature reaches 165°F (74°C).
6. Let the meatloaf rest for 10 minutes before slicing and serving.

Nutrition Info (per serving):

- Calories: 300
- Protein: 28g
- Carbohydrates: 12g
- Fiber: 2g
- Sugars: 2g
- Fat: 16g
- Saturated Fat: 4g

Serves: 4

Cooking Time: 55 minutes

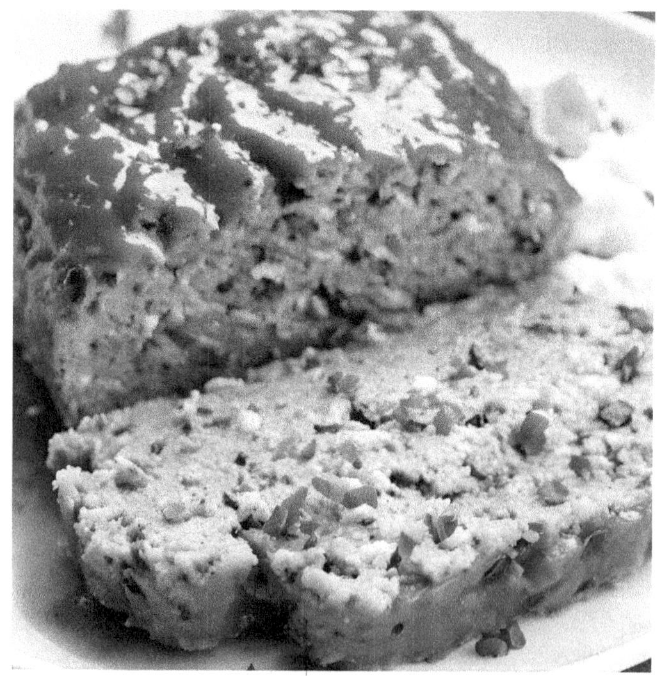

25. Szechuan Chicken Stir Fry

Ingredients:

- 1 pound boneless, skinless chicken breasts, thinly sliced
- 2 tablespoons sesame oil
- 2 cloves garlic, minced
- 1 tablespoon grated ginger
- 1 red bell pepper, sliced
- 1 green bell pepper, sliced
- 1 cup snap peas
- 2 tablespoons low-sodium soy sauce
- 1 tablespoon rice vinegar
- 1 tablespoon chili paste (adjust to taste)
- 1 tablespoon honey
- 1/4 cup chopped green onions

Instructions:

1. Heat 1 tablespoon of sesame oil in a large skillet or wok over medium-high heat.
2. Add the chicken slices and cook until browned and cooked through, about 5-7 minutes. Remove the chicken from the skillet and set aside.
3. Add the remaining sesame oil to the skillet. Add the minced garlic and grated ginger, cooking for 1 minute until fragrant.
4. Add the red bell pepper, green bell pepper, and snap peas. Stir-fry for 5-7 minutes until the vegetables are tender-crisp.
5. Return the chicken to the skillet.
6. In a small bowl, mix the soy sauce, rice vinegar, chili paste, and honey. Pour the sauce over the chicken and vegetables, stirring to coat evenly.
7. Cook for another 2-3 minutes until everything is heated through.
8. Garnish with chopped green onions before serving.
9. Serve immediately.

Nutrition Info (per serving):

- Calories: 260
- Protein: 26g
- Carbohydrates: 14g
- Fiber: 3g
- Sugars: 7g
- Fat: 12g
- Saturated Fat: 2g

Serves: 4

Cooking Time: 25 minutes

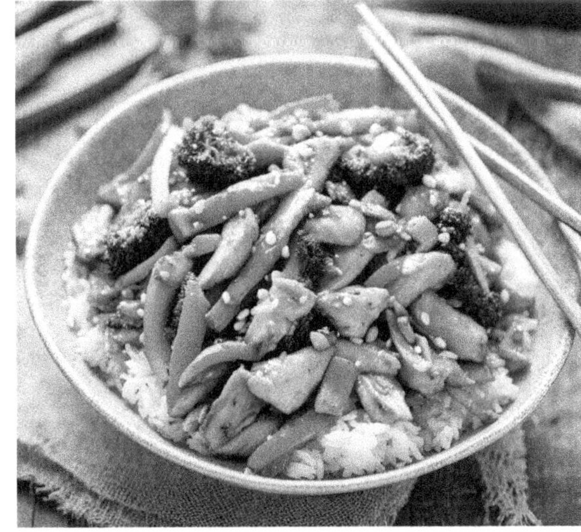

26. Chicken and Mushroom Crepes

Ingredients:

- 1 pound boneless, skinless chicken breasts, thinly sliced
- 2 tablespoons olive oil
- 1 large onion, chopped
- 2 cloves garlic, minced
- 2 cups sliced mushrooms (any variety)
- 1 cup low-fat milk
- 1/2 cup low-fat Greek yogurt
- 1/4 cup grated Parmesan cheese
- 1 teaspoon dried thyme
- 8 whole grain crepes (store-bought or homemade)

Instructions:

1. Heat 1 tablespoon of olive oil in a large skillet over medium-high heat. Add the chicken slices and cook until browned and cooked through, about 5-7 minutes. Remove the chicken from the skillet and set aside.
2. Add the remaining olive oil to the skillet. Add the chopped onion and minced garlic, cooking for 3-4 minutes until softened.
3. Add the sliced mushrooms and cook for another 5-7 minutes until tender.
4. Stir in the milk, Greek yogurt, Parmesan cheese, and dried thyme. Cook for 3-4 minutes until the sauce thickens.
5. Return the chicken to the skillet and toss to coat in the sauce.
6. Fill each crepe with the chicken and mushroom mixture.
7. Serve hot.

Nutrition Info (per serving):

- Calories: 320
- Protein: 25g
- Carbohydrates: 28g
- Fiber: 4g
- Sugars: 7g
- Fat: 12g
- Saturated Fat: 3g

Serves: 4
Cooking Time: 30 minutes

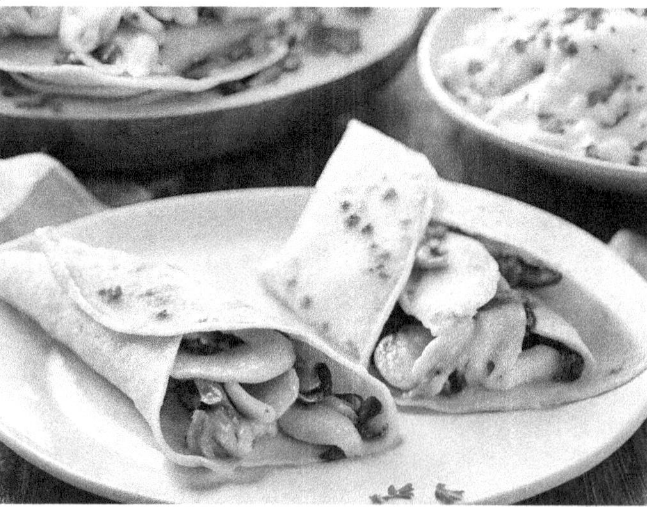

27. Chicken Ratatouille

Ingredients:

- 2 tablespoons olive oil
- 1 pound boneless, skinless chicken thighs, cut into chunks
- 1 large onion, chopped
- 3 cloves garlic, minced
- 1 eggplant, cubed
- 2 zucchinis, sliced
- 1 red bell pepper, chopped
- 1 yellow bell pepper, chopped
- 2 cups chopped tomatoes
- 1 teaspoon dried basil
- 1 teaspoon dried oregano
- 1/4 cup chopped fresh parsley

Instructions:

1. Heat 1 tablespoon of olive oil in a large pot over medium-high heat. Add the chicken chunks and cook until browned, about 5-7 minutes. Remove the chicken from the pot and set aside.
2. Add the remaining olive oil to the pot. Add the chopped onion and minced garlic, cooking for 3-4 minutes until softened.
3. Stir in the eggplant, zucchinis, red bell pepper, and yellow bell pepper. Cook for 5-7 minutes until the vegetables are tender.
4. Add the chopped tomatoes, dried basil, and dried oregano. Cook for another 10 minutes.
5. Return the chicken to the pot and simmer for 10-15 minutes until the chicken is cooked through and the flavors are well combined.
6. Stir in the chopped fresh parsley before serving.
7. Serve hot.

Nutrition Info (per serving):

- Calories: 280
- Protein: 24g
- Carbohydrates: 18g
- Fiber: 6g
- Sugars: 9g
- Fat: 14g
- Saturated Fat: 3g

Serves: 4

Cooking Time: 40 minutes

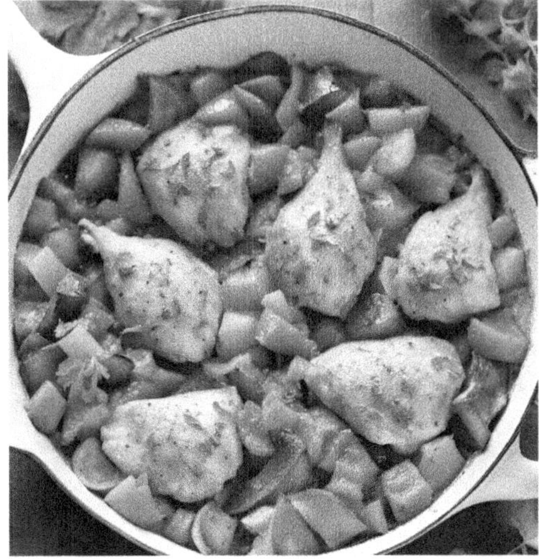

Fish & Seafood Recipes

1. Grilled Salmon with Dill and Lemon
Ingredients:

- 4 salmon fillets (6 ounces each)
- 2 tablespoons olive oil
- 2 tablespoons fresh dill, chopped
- 1 lemon, thinly sliced
- 1 tablespoon lemon juice
- 2 cloves garlic, minced

Instructions:

1. Preheat the grill to medium-high heat.
2. In a small bowl, mix the olive oil, chopped dill, lemon juice, and minced garlic.
3. Brush the mixture over the salmon fillets.
4. Place the lemon slices on top of each fillet.
5. Grill the salmon fillets for 4-5 minutes per side, until the fish flakes easily with a fork.
6. Serve hot.

Nutrition Info (per serving):

- Calories: 300
- Protein: 34g
- Carbohydrates: 2g
- Fiber: 0g
- Sugars: 0g
- Fat: 18g
- Saturated Fat: 3g

Serves: 4
Cooking Time: 15 minutes

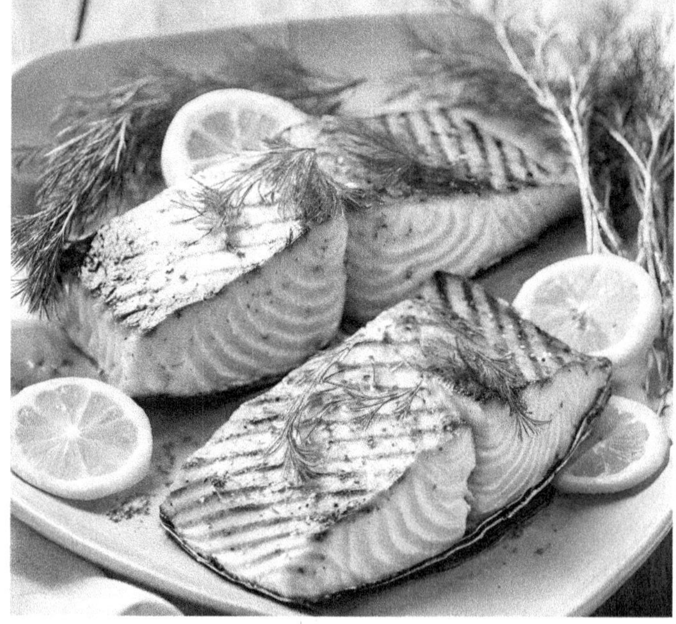

2. Baked Cod with Cherry Tomatoes

Ingredients:

- 4 cod fillets (6 ounces each)
- 2 tablespoons olive oil
- 1 pint cherry tomatoes, halved
- 3 cloves garlic, minced
- 1 tablespoon fresh basil, chopped
- 1 teaspoon dried oregano
- 1 lemon, thinly sliced

Instructions:

1. Preheat the oven to 375°F (190°C).
2. Place the cod fillets in a baking dish.
3. In a small bowl, mix the olive oil, minced garlic, chopped basil, and dried oregano.
4. Pour the mixture over the cod fillets.
5. Arrange the cherry tomatoes and lemon slices around the cod.
6. Bake in the preheated oven for 20-25 minutes, until the fish is opaque and flakes easily with a fork.
7. Serve hot.

Nutrition Info (per serving):

- Calories: 200
- Protein: 28g
- Carbohydrates: 5g
- Fiber: 1g
- Sugars: 3g
- Fat: 8g
- Saturated Fat: 1g

Serves: 4
Cooking Time: 30 minutes

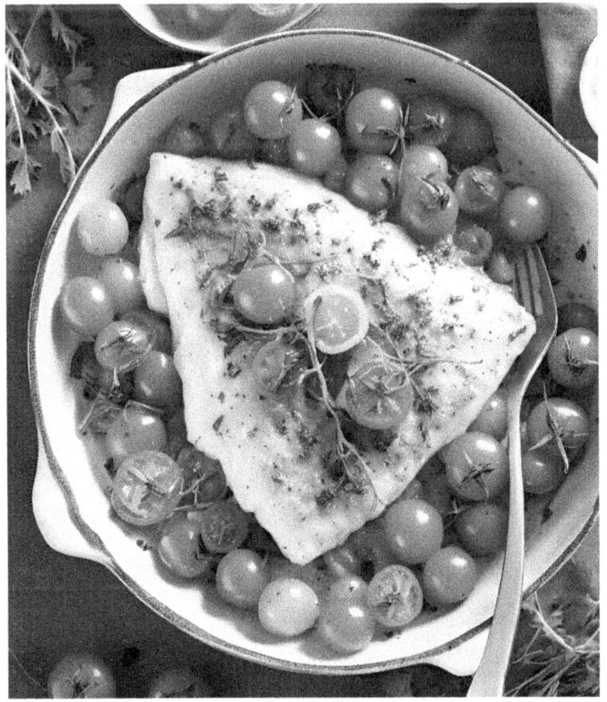

3. Seared Tuna Steaks

Ingredients:

- 4 tuna steaks (6 ounces each)
- 2 tablespoons olive oil
- 2 tablespoons low-sodium soy sauce
- 1 tablespoon lemon juice
- 1 tablespoon grated ginger
- 2 cloves garlic, minced

Instructions:

1. In a small bowl, mix the olive oil, soy sauce, lemon juice, grated ginger, and minced garlic.
2. Brush the mixture over the tuna steaks.
3. Heat a skillet over high heat.
4. Sear the tuna steaks for 1-2 minutes per side, until the outside is browned but the inside is still pink.
5. Serve hot.

Nutrition Info (per serving):

- Calories: 250
- Protein: 34g
- Carbohydrates: 1g
- Fiber: 0g
- Sugars: 0g
- Fat: 12g
- Saturated Fat: 2g

Serves: 4

Cooking Time: 10 minutes

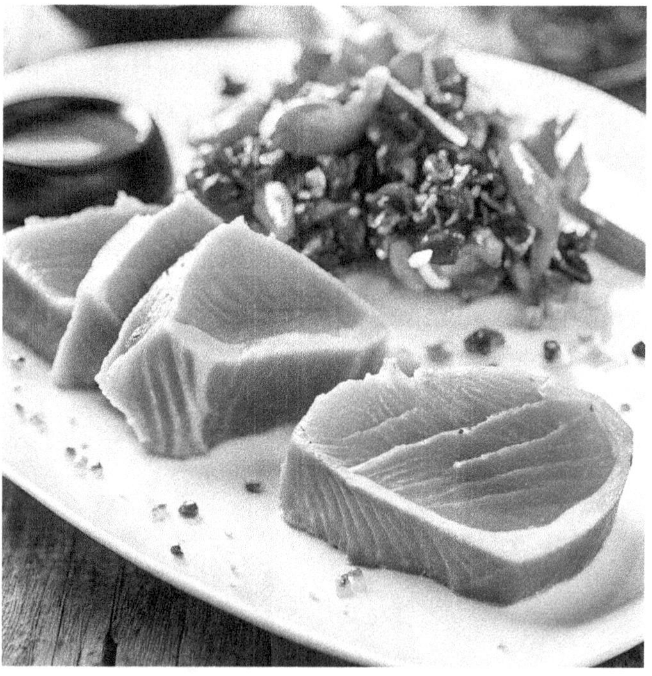

4. Herb-Crusted Tilapia

Ingredients:

- 4 tilapia fillets (6 ounces each)
- 1/2 cup whole grain breadcrumbs
- 1/4 cup grated Parmesan cheese
- 2 tablespoons fresh parsley, chopped
- 1 tablespoon fresh thyme, chopped
- 2 cloves garlic, minced
- 2 tablespoons olive oil

Instructions:

1. Preheat the oven to 400°F (200°C).
2. In a small bowl, mix the breadcrumbs, Parmesan cheese, chopped parsley, chopped thyme, and minced garlic.
3. Brush the tilapia fillets with olive oil.
4. Press the breadcrumb mixture onto the fillets.
5. Place the fillets on a baking sheet.
6. Bake in the preheated oven for 12-15 minutes, until the fish is opaque and flakes easily with a fork.
7. Serve hot.

Nutrition Info (per serving):

- Calories: 260
- Protein: 34g
- Carbohydrates: 10g
- Fiber: 1g
- Sugars: 1g
- Fat: 10g
- Saturated Fat: 2g

Serves: 4
Cooking Time: 20 minutes

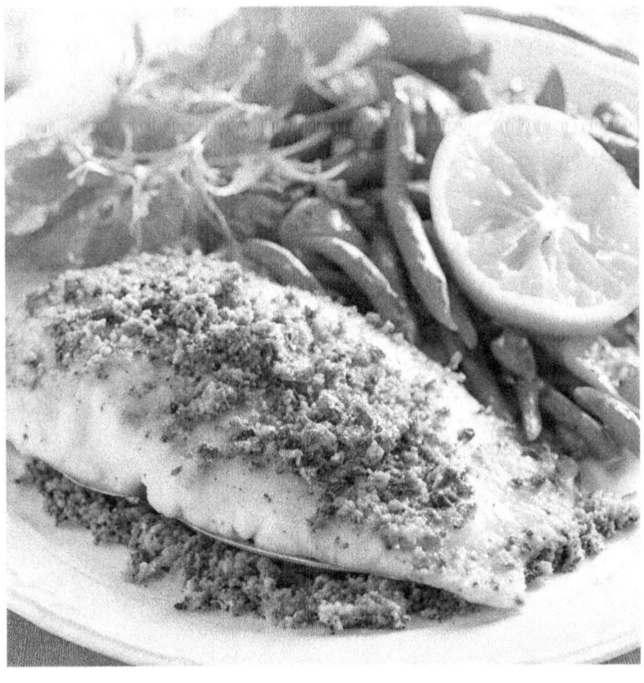

5. Fisherman's Stew

Ingredients:

- 2 tablespoons olive oil
- 1 large onion, chopped
- 3 cloves garlic, minced
- 1 red bell pepper, chopped
- 1 yellow bell pepper, chopped
- 1 can (14.5 oz) diced tomatoes, no salt added
- 4 cups low-sodium fish or vegetable broth
- 1 pound white fish fillets (such as cod or halibut), cut into chunks
- 1/2 pound shrimp, peeled and deveined
- 1/2 pound mussels, cleaned and debearded
- 1 teaspoon dried thyme
- 1 teaspoon paprika
- 1/4 cup chopped fresh parsley
- 1 lemon, cut into wedges

Instructions:

1. Heat the olive oil in a large pot over medium heat.
2. Add the chopped onion, garlic, and bell peppers, cooking for 5-7 minutes until softened.
3. Stir in the diced tomatoes, fish broth, thyme, and paprika. Bring to a boil.
4. Reduce heat and simmer for 10 minutes.
5. Add the fish chunks, shrimp, and mussels to the pot. Simmer for another 5-7 minutes until the fish is opaque and the mussels have opened.
6. Stir in the chopped fresh parsley before serving.
7. Serve hot with lemon wedges.

Nutrition Info (per serving):

- Calories: 280
- Protein: 35g
- Carbohydrates: 12g
- Fiber: 3g
- Sugars: 5g
- Fat: 10g
- Saturated Fat: 1.5g

Serves: 4

Cooking Time: 30 minutes

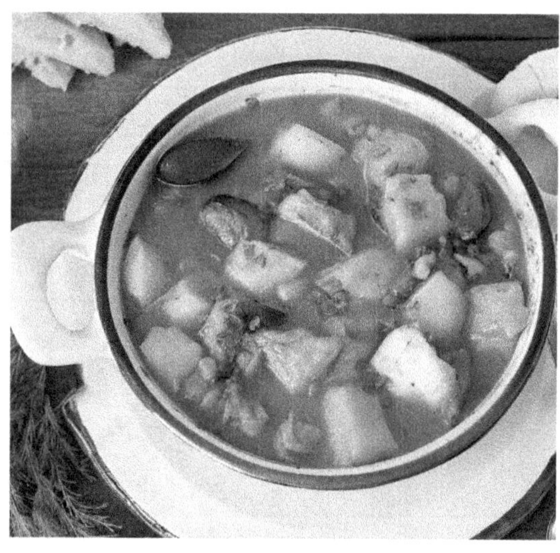

6. Seafood Gumbo

Ingredients:

- 2 tablespoons olive oil
- 1/4 cup whole grain flour
- 1 large onion, chopped
- 1 green bell pepper, chopped
- 2 celery stalks, chopped
- 3 cloves garlic, minced
- 1 can (14.5 oz) diced tomatoes, no salt added
- 4 cups low-sodium chicken broth
- 1 pound shrimp, peeled and deveined
- 1/2 pound crabmeat
- 1/2 pound white fish fillets, cut into chunks
- 1 teaspoon dried thyme
- 1 teaspoon paprika
- 1 teaspoon filé powder (optional)
- 1/4 cup chopped fresh parsley

Instructions:

1. Heat the olive oil in a large pot over medium heat.
2. Whisk in the flour and cook for 5-7 minutes, stirring constantly, until the roux is golden brown.
3. Add the chopped onion, bell pepper, celery, and garlic. Cook for another 5-7 minutes until softened.
4. Stir in the diced tomatoes, chicken broth, thyme, and paprika. Bring to a boil.
5. Reduce heat and simmer for 15 minutes.
6. Add the shrimp, crabmeat, and fish chunks. Simmer for another 5-7 minutes until the seafood is cooked through.
7. Stir in the filé powder (if using) and chopped fresh parsley before serving.
8. Serve hot.

Nutrition Info (per serving):

- Calories: 320
- Protein: 32g
- Carbohydrates: 18g
- Fiber: 3g
- Sugars: 6g
- Fat: 12g
- Saturated Fat: 2g

Serves: 4
Cooking Time: 45 minutes

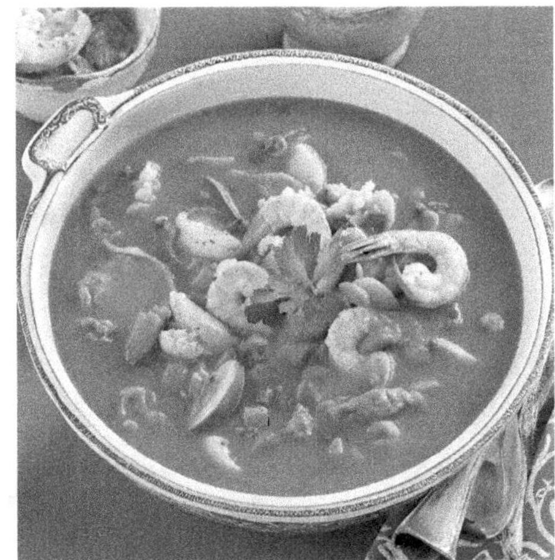

7. Mediterranean Fish Soup

Ingredients:

- 2 tablespoons olive oil
- 1 large onion, chopped
- 3 cloves garlic, minced
- 2 cups diced tomatoes, no salt added
- 4 cups low-sodium vegetable broth
- 1 cup water
- 1/2 cup white wine (optional)
- 1 teaspoon dried oregano
- 1 teaspoon dried basil
- 1/2 teaspoon paprika
- 1 pound white fish fillets (such as cod or halibut), cut into chunks
- 1/2 pound shrimp, peeled and deveined
- 1/4 cup chopped fresh parsley
- 1 lemon, cut into wedges

Instructions:

1. Heat the olive oil in a large pot over medium heat.
2. Add the chopped onion and garlic, cooking for 5-7 minutes until softened.
3. Stir in the diced tomatoes, vegetable broth, water, white wine (if using), oregano, basil, and paprika. Bring to a boil.
4. Reduce heat and simmer for 10 minutes.
5. Add the fish chunks and shrimp to the pot. Simmer for another 5-7 minutes until the seafood is cooked through.
6. Stir in the chopped fresh parsley before serving.
7. Serve hot with lemon wedges.

Nutrition Info (per serving):

- Calories: 260
- Protein: 30g
- Carbohydrates: 10g
- Fiber: 3g
- Sugars: 5g
- Fat: 10g
- Saturated Fat: 1.5g

Serves: 4

Cooking Time: 30 minutes

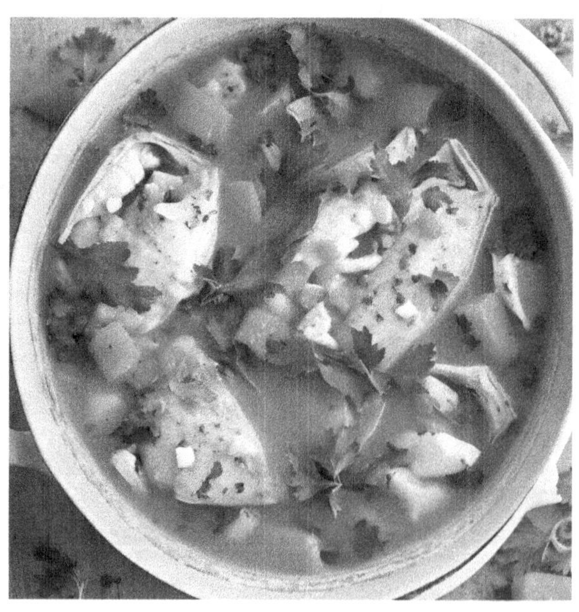

8. Shrimp Risotto

Ingredients:

- 2 tablespoons olive oil
- 1 large onion, chopped
- 2 cloves garlic, minced
- 1 cup Arborio rice
- 1/2 cup white wine (optional)
- 4 cups low-sodium chicken broth, warmed
- 1 pound shrimp, peeled and deveined
- 1/2 cup grated Parmesan cheese
- 1 tablespoon lemon juice
- 1/4 cup chopped fresh parsley

Instructions:

1. Heat the olive oil in a large pot over medium heat.
2. Add the chopped onion and garlic, cooking for 5-7 minutes until softened.
3. Stir in the Arborio rice and cook for 1-2 minutes until lightly toasted.
4. Pour in the white wine (if using) and cook until absorbed.
5. Gradually add the warm chicken broth, one ladleful at a time, stirring constantly until absorbed before adding more. Continue until the rice is creamy and cooked through, about 18-20 minutes.
6. Stir in the shrimp and cook for 3-4 minutes until pink and cooked through.
7. Remove from heat and stir in the Parmesan cheese, lemon juice, and chopped fresh parsley.
8. Serve hot.

Nutrition Info (per serving):

- Calories: 350
- Protein: 28g
- Carbohydrates: 40g
- Fiber: 2g
- Sugars: 4g
- Fat: 10g
- Saturated Fat: 3g

Serves: 4
Cooking Time: 30 minutes

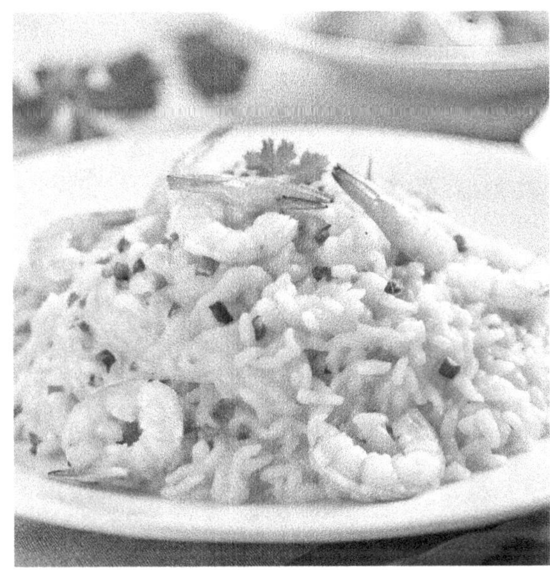

9. Salmon and Pea Tagliatelle

Ingredients:

- 8 ounces whole grain tagliatelle
- 1 tablespoon olive oil
- 1 pound salmon fillets, skin removed and cut into chunks
- 2 cloves garlic, minced
- 1 cup frozen peas, thawed
- 1/2 cup low-fat Greek yogurt
- 1/4 cup grated Parmesan cheese
- 1 tablespoon lemon juice
- 1 teaspoon lemon zest
- 1/4 cup chopped fresh dill

Instructions:

1. Cook the tagliatelle according to package instructions. Drain and set aside.
2. Heat the olive oil in a large skillet over medium-high heat. Add the salmon chunks and cook for 3-4 minutes until browned and cooked through. Remove from the skillet and set aside.
3. Add the minced garlic to the skillet and cook for 1 minute until fragrant.
4. Stir in the peas and cook for another 2 minutes.
5. Reduce heat to low and stir in the Greek yogurt, Parmesan cheese, lemon juice, and lemon zest. Cook for 2-3 minutes until heated through.
6. Return the salmon to the skillet and toss to coat in the sauce.
7. Serve the salmon and pea mixture over the cooked tagliatelle, garnished with chopped fresh dill.
8. Serve hot.

Nutrition Info (per serving):

- Calories: 380
- Protein: 30g
- Carbohydrates: 40g
- Fiber: 6g
- Sugars: 4g
- Fat: 12g
- Saturated Fat: 3g

Serves: 4

Cooking Time: 25 minutes

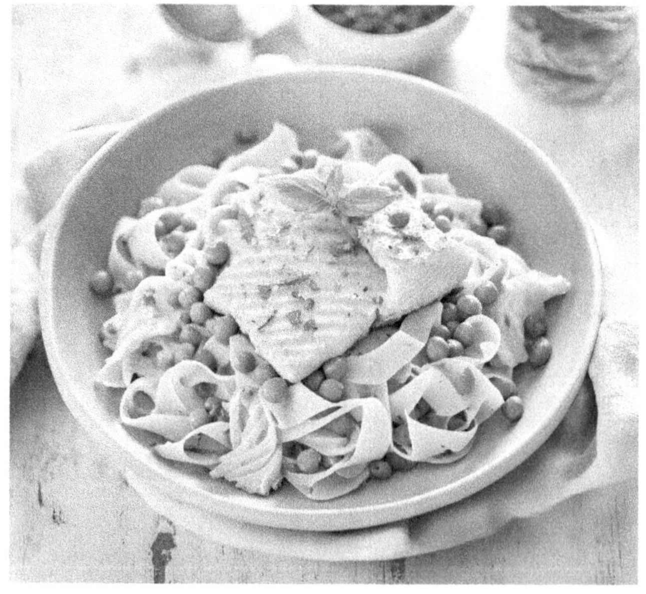

10. Barbecue Glazed Salmon

Ingredients:
- 4 salmon fillets (6 ounces each)
- 1/2 cup barbecue sauce (low-sugar)
- 1 tablespoon olive oil
- 1 tablespoon lemon juice
- 1 teaspoon smoked paprika
- 2 cloves garlic, minced

Instructions:
1. Preheat the oven to 375°F (190°C).
2. In a small bowl, mix the barbecue sauce, olive oil, lemon juice, smoked paprika, and minced garlic.
3. Place the salmon fillets on a baking sheet lined with parchment paper.
4. Brush the barbecue mixture over the salmon fillets.
5. Bake in the preheated oven for 15-20 minutes until the fish flakes easily with a fork.
6. Serve hot.

Nutrition Info (per serving):
- Calories: 320
- Protein: 34g
- Carbohydrates: 10g
- Fiber: 1g
- Sugars: 6g
- Fat: 16g
- Saturated Fat: 3g

Serves: 4
Cooking Time: 20 minutes

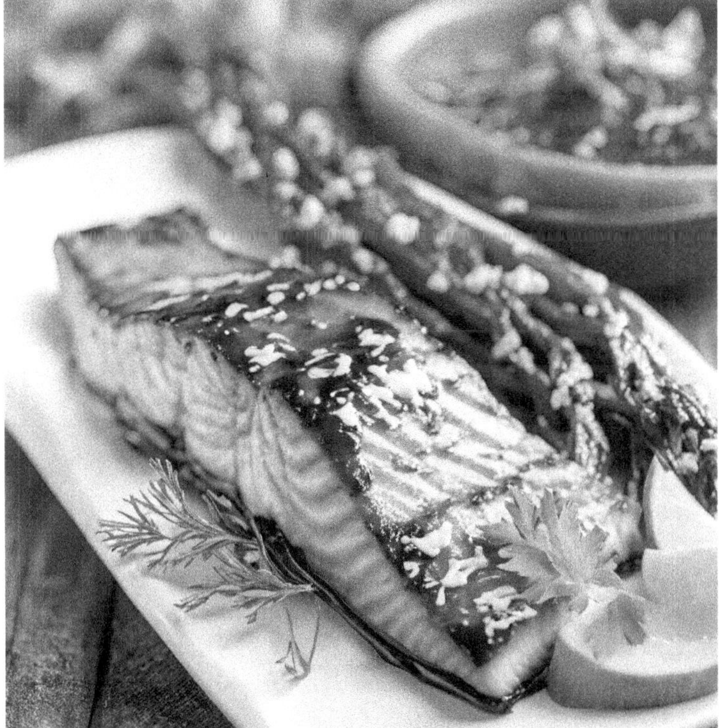

11. Grilled Shrimp Skewers

Ingredients:

- 1 pound large shrimp, peeled and deveined
- 2 tablespoons olive oil
- 1 tablespoon lemon juice
- 2 cloves garlic, minced
- 1 teaspoon dried oregano
- 1 teaspoon smoked paprika
- Wooden skewers, soaked in water for 30 minutes

Instructions:

1. Preheat the grill to medium-high heat.
2. In a large bowl, mix the olive oil, lemon juice, minced garlic, dried oregano, and smoked paprika.
3. Add the shrimp to the bowl and toss to coat evenly.
4. Thread the shrimp onto the soaked wooden skewers.
5. Grill the shrimp skewers for 2-3 minutes per side until the shrimp are pink and cooked through.
6. Serve hot.

Nutrition Info (per serving):

- Calories: 200
- Protein: 26g
- Carbohydrates: 2g
- Fiber: 0g
- Sugars: 0g
- Fat: 10g
- Saturated Fat: 2g

Serves: 4

Cooking Time: 10 minutes

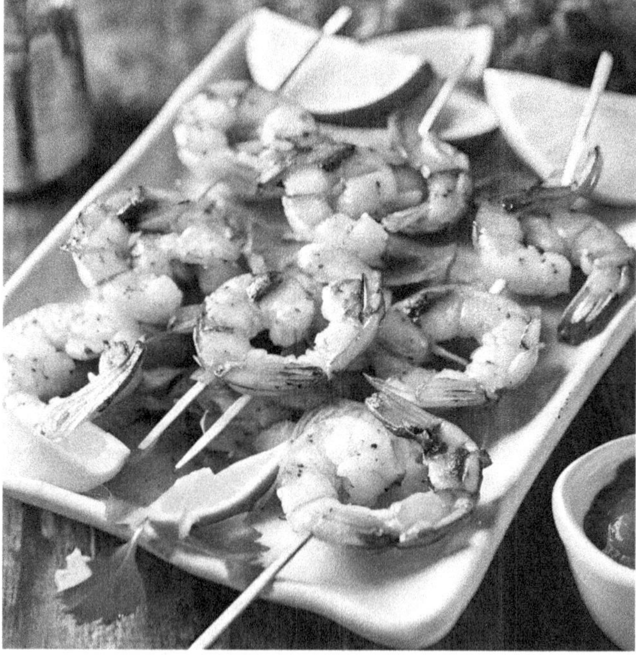

12. Swordfish Steaks with Cilantro Lime Butter

Ingredients:

- 4 swordfish steaks (6 ounces each)
- 2 tablespoons olive oil
- 1 tablespoon lime juice
- 1/4 cup unsalted butter, softened
- 2 tablespoons chopped fresh cilantro
- 1 clove garlic, minced
- 1 teaspoon lime zest

Instructions:

1. Preheat the grill to medium-high heat.
2. In a small bowl, mix the olive oil and lime juice.
3. Brush the mixture over the swordfish steaks.
4. Grill the swordfish steaks for 4-5 minutes per side until cooked through.
5. In another small bowl, mix the softened butter, chopped cilantro, minced garlic, and lime zest.
6. Serve the grilled swordfish steaks topped with the cilantro lime butter.

Nutrition Info (per serving):

- Calories: 380
- Protein: 36g
- Carbohydrates: 2g
- Fiber: 0g
- Sugars: 0g
- Fat: 24g
- Saturated Fat: 10g

Serves: 4

Cooking Time: 15 minutes

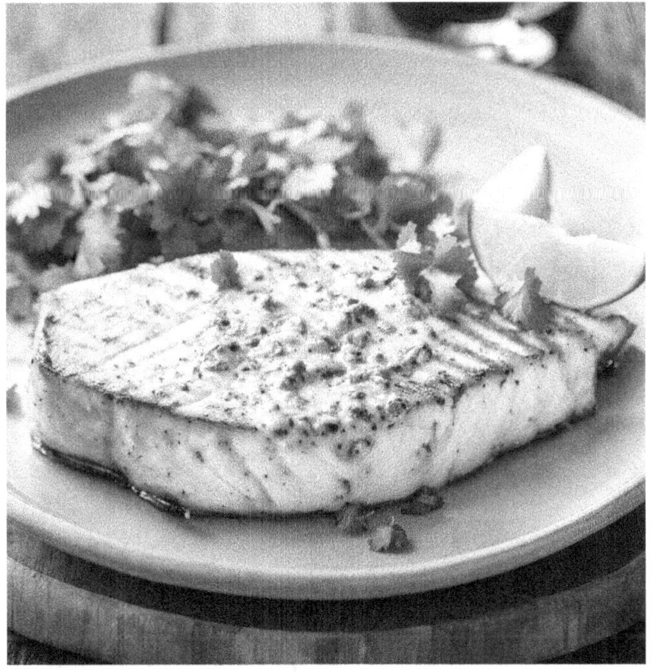

13. Miso Glazed Cod

Ingredients:

- 4 cod fillets (6 ounces each)
- 1/4 cup white miso paste
- 2 tablespoons mirin (sweet rice wine)
- 2 tablespoons sake (Japanese rice wine)
- 1 tablespoon honey
- 1 tablespoon rice vinegar
- 1 tablespoon olive oil

Instructions:

1. In a small bowl, mix the miso paste, mirin, sake, honey, rice vinegar, and olive oil until smooth.
2. Place the cod fillets in a shallow dish and pour the miso mixture over them. Marinate in the refrigerator for 30 minutes.
3. Preheat the oven to 400°F (200°C).
4. Place the marinated cod fillets on a baking sheet lined with parchment paper.
5. Bake in the preheated oven for 12-15 minutes until the fish flakes easily with a fork.
6. Serve hot.

Nutrition Info (per serving):

- Calories: 280
- Protein: 32g
- Carbohydrates: 8g
- Fiber: 0g
- Sugars: 6g
- Fat: 12g
- Saturated Fat: 2g

Serves: 4

Cooking Time: 45 minutes (including marinating time)

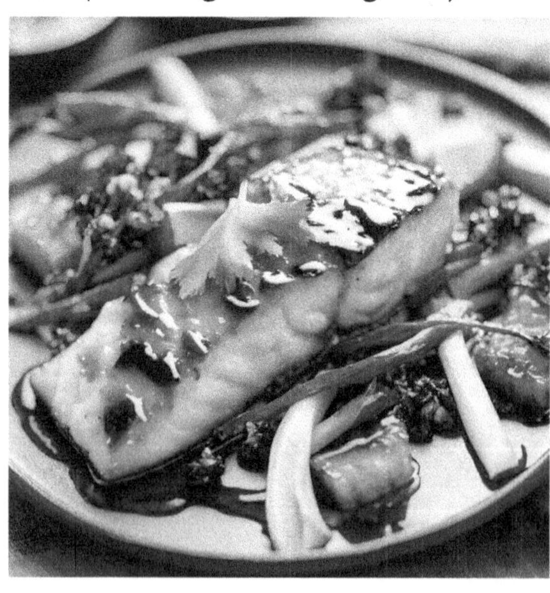

14. Vietnamese Fish Tacos

Ingredients:

- 1 pound white fish fillets (such as tilapia or cod), cut into strips
- 2 tablespoons olive oil
- 1 tablespoon lime juice
- 1 tablespoon fish sauce
- 1 teaspoon grated ginger
- 1 clove garlic, minced
- 8 small corn tortillas
- 1 cup shredded cabbage
- 1/2 cup grated carrots
- 1/4 cup chopped fresh cilantro
- 1 tablespoon sriracha sauce (optional)
- 1 lime, cut into wedges

Instructions:

1. In a large bowl, mix the olive oil, lime juice, fish sauce, grated ginger, and minced garlic.
2. Add the fish strips to the bowl and toss to coat evenly. Marinate in the refrigerator for 15 minutes.
3. Preheat a grill or grill pan to medium-high heat.
4. Grill the fish strips for 2-3 minutes per side until cooked through.
5. Warm the corn tortillas on the grill for about 30 seconds per side.
6. Assemble the tacos by placing the grilled fish on the tortillas, topped with shredded cabbage, grated carrots, and chopped cilantro.
7. Drizzle with sriracha sauce (if using) and serve with lime wedges.
8. Serve immediately.

Nutrition Info (per serving):

- Calories: 280
- Protein: 24g
- Carbohydrates: 20g
- Fiber: 4g
- Sugars: 2g
- Fat: 12g
- Saturated Fat: 2g

Serves: 4
Cooking Time: 25 minutes

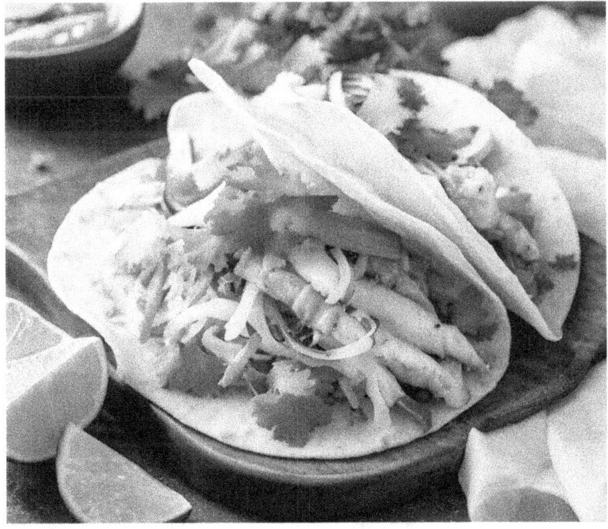

15. Korean Grilled Mackerel

Ingredients:

- 4 mackerel fillets
- 2 tablespoons soy sauce (low-sodium)
- 1 tablespoon sesame oil
- 1 tablespoon rice vinegar
- 1 tablespoon honey
- 2 cloves garlic, minced
- 1 teaspoon grated ginger
- 1 tablespoon sesame seeds
- 2 green onions, chopped

Instructions:

1. In a small bowl, mix the soy sauce, sesame oil, rice vinegar, honey, minced garlic, and grated ginger.
2. Place the mackerel fillets in a shallow dish and pour the marinade over them. Let marinate in the refrigerator for 20 minutes.
3. Preheat the grill to medium-high heat.
4. Remove the mackerel from the marinade and grill for 3-4 minutes on each side until cooked through.
5. Sprinkle with sesame seeds and chopped green onions before serving.
6. Serve hot.

Nutrition Info (per serving):

- Calories: 280
- Protein: 28g
- Carbohydrates: 5g
- Fiber: 1g
- Sugars: 3g
- Fat: 16g
- Saturated Fat: 4g

Serves: 4

Cooking Time: 25 minutes (including marinating time)

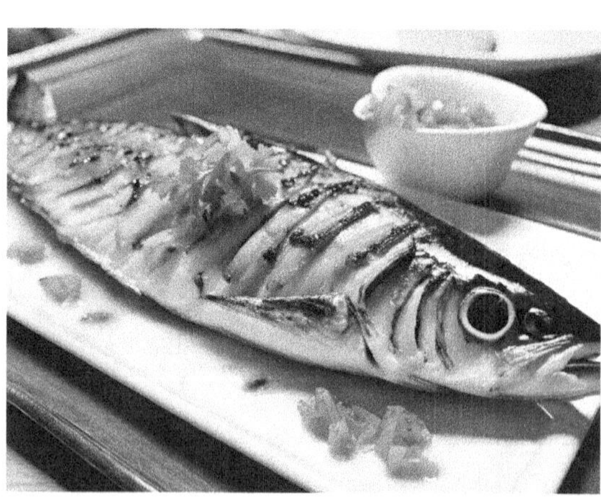

16. Shrimp Caesar Salad

Ingredients:

- 1 pound shrimp, peeled and deveined
- 2 tablespoons olive oil
- 1 teaspoon garlic powder
- 1 large romaine lettuce, chopped
- 1/4 cup grated Parmesan cheese
- 1/4 cup Caesar dressing (low-fat)
- 1 cup whole grain croutons
- 1 lemon, cut into wedges

Instructions:

1. Preheat a grill or grill pan to medium-high heat.
2. In a bowl, toss the shrimp with olive oil and garlic powder.
3. Grill the shrimp for 2-3 minutes on each side until pink and cooked through. Set aside.
4. In a large bowl, combine the chopped romaine lettuce, grated Parmesan cheese, and Caesar dressing. Toss to coat.
5. Top the salad with the grilled shrimp and whole grain croutons.
6. Serve with lemon wedges.
7. Serve immediately.

Nutrition Info (per serving):

- Calories: 320
- Protein: 28g
- Carbohydrates: 16g
- Fiber: 4g
- Sugars: 2g
- Fat: 16g
- Saturated Fat: 3g

Serves: 4

Cooking Time: 15 minutes

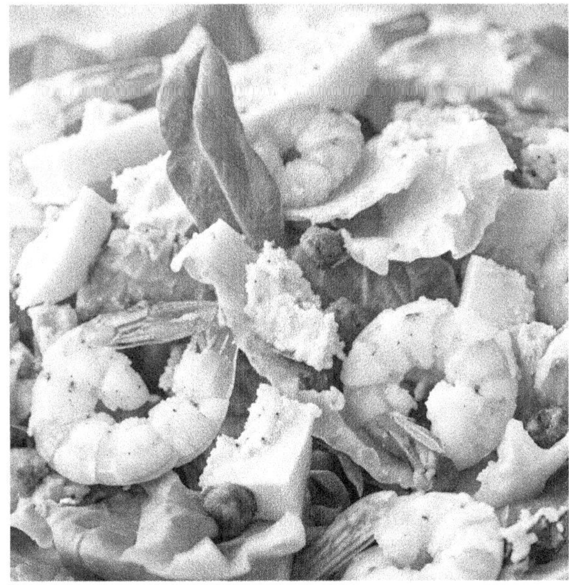

17. Tuna Salad Stuffed Tomatoes

Ingredients:

- 4 large tomatoes
- 2 cans (5 oz each) tuna in water, drained
- 1/4 cup low-fat Greek yogurt
- 1 tablespoon Dijon mustard
- 1/4 cup finely chopped celery
- 1/4 cup finely chopped red onion
- 1 tablespoon lemon juice
- 1 tablespoon chopped fresh parsley

Instructions:

1. Cut the tops off the tomatoes and scoop out the seeds and pulp.
2. In a medium bowl, combine the drained tuna, Greek yogurt, Dijon mustard, chopped celery, chopped red onion, lemon juice, and chopped parsley. Mix well.
3. Spoon the tuna mixture into the hollowed-out tomatoes.
4. Serve immediately or refrigerate for later.

Nutrition Info (per serving):

- Calories: 150
- Protein: 18g
- Carbohydrates: 8g
- Fiber: 2g
- Sugars: 5g
- Fat: 5g
- Saturated Fat: 1g

Serves: 4
Cooking Time: 15 minutes

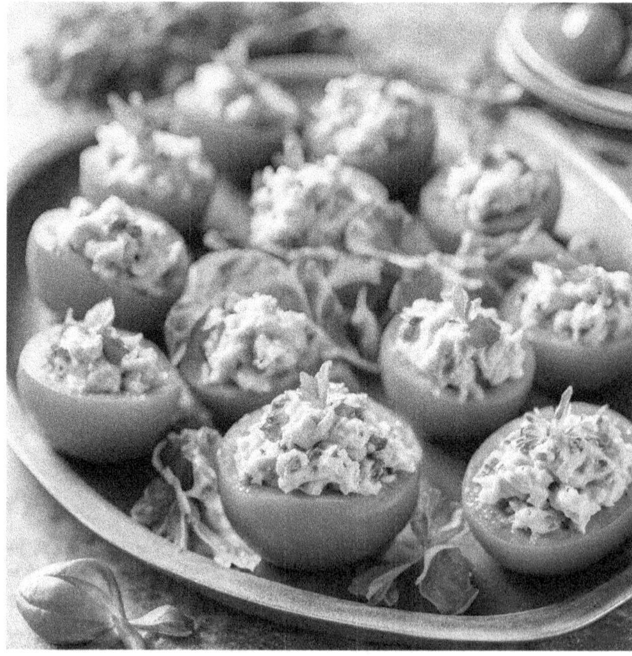

18. Seared Scallop Salad

Ingredients:

- 1 pound large sea scallops
- 2 tablespoons olive oil
- 1 teaspoon garlic powder
- 6 cups mixed salad greens
- 1 cup cherry tomatoes, halved
- 1 avocado, sliced
- 1/4 cup chopped red onion
- 1/4 cup balsamic vinaigrette (low-fat)

Instructions:

1. Pat the scallops dry with a paper towel and season with garlic powder.
2. Heat the olive oil in a large skillet over medium-high heat.
3. Add the scallops to the skillet and sear for 2-3 minutes on each side until golden brown and cooked through. Remove from heat.
4. In a large bowl, combine the mixed salad greens, cherry tomatoes, avocado slices, and chopped red onion.
5. Top the salad with the seared scallops.
6. Drizzle with balsamic vinaigrette before serving.
7. Serve immediately.

Nutrition Info (per serving):

- Calories: 280
- Protein: 22g
- Carbohydrates: 14g
- Fiber: 6g
- Sugars: 5g
- Fat: 10g
- Saturated Fat: 2g

Serves: 4
Cooking Time: 15 minutes

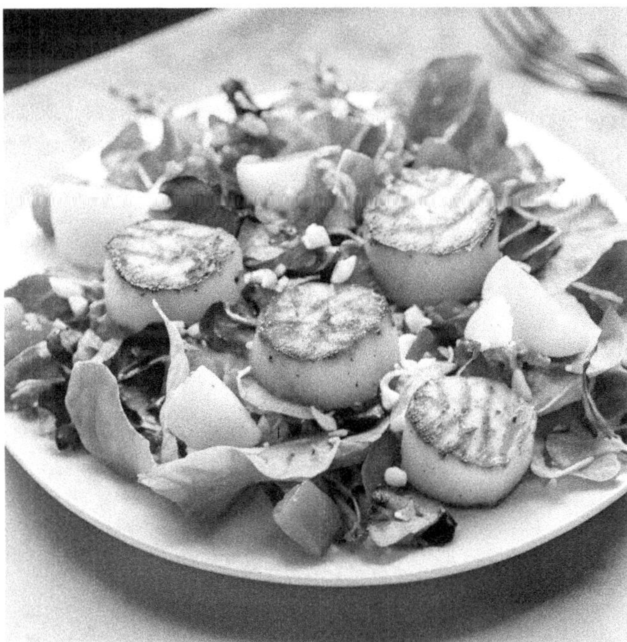

19. Broiled Scallops with Parmesan Crust

Ingredients:

- 1 pound large sea scallops
- 2 tablespoons olive oil
- 1/2 cup grated Parmesan cheese
- 1/4 cup whole grain breadcrumbs
- 2 cloves garlic, minced
- 1 teaspoon dried thyme
- 1 tablespoon lemon juice

Instructions:

1. Preheat the broiler on high.
2. Pat the scallops dry with a paper towel and place them in a baking dish.
3. In a small bowl, mix the olive oil, Parmesan cheese, breadcrumbs, minced garlic, and dried thyme.
4. Spoon the mixture evenly over the scallops.
5. Broil the scallops for 6-8 minutes, until the tops are golden and the scallops are cooked through.
6. Drizzle with lemon juice before serving.
7. Serve hot.

Nutrition Info (per serving):

- Calories: 280
- Protein: 22g
- Carbohydrates: 6g
- Fiber: 1g
- Sugars: 1g
- Fat: 18g
- Saturated Fat: 5g

Serves: 4

Cooking Time: 15 minutes

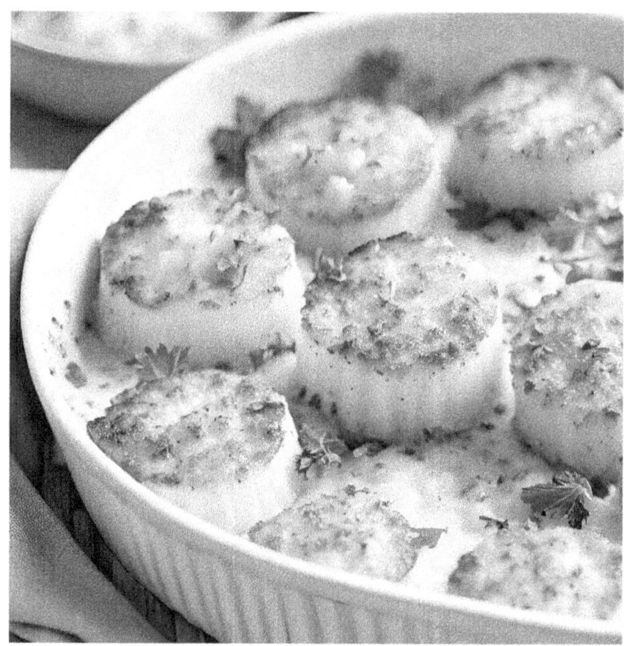

20. Pesto Baked Salmon

Ingredients:

- 4 salmon fillets (6 ounces each)
- 1/2 cup homemade or store-bought pesto (without cheese for a vegan option)
- 1 tablespoon olive oil
- 1 lemon, thinly sliced
- 1/4 cup pine nuts (optional)

Instructions:

1. Preheat the oven to 375°F (190°C).
2. Place the salmon fillets on a baking sheet lined with parchment paper.
3. Spread the pesto evenly over the salmon fillets.
4. Arrange the lemon slices on top of the pesto.
5. Drizzle with olive oil and sprinkle with pine nuts if using.
6. Bake in the preheated oven for 15-20 minutes until the salmon is cooked through and flakes easily with a fork.
7. Serve hot.

Nutrition Info (per serving):

- Calories: 350
- Protein: 34g
- Carbohydrates: 3g
- Fiber: 1g
- Sugars: 1g
- Fat: 22g
- Saturated Fat: 4g

Serves: 4
Cooking Time: 20 minutes

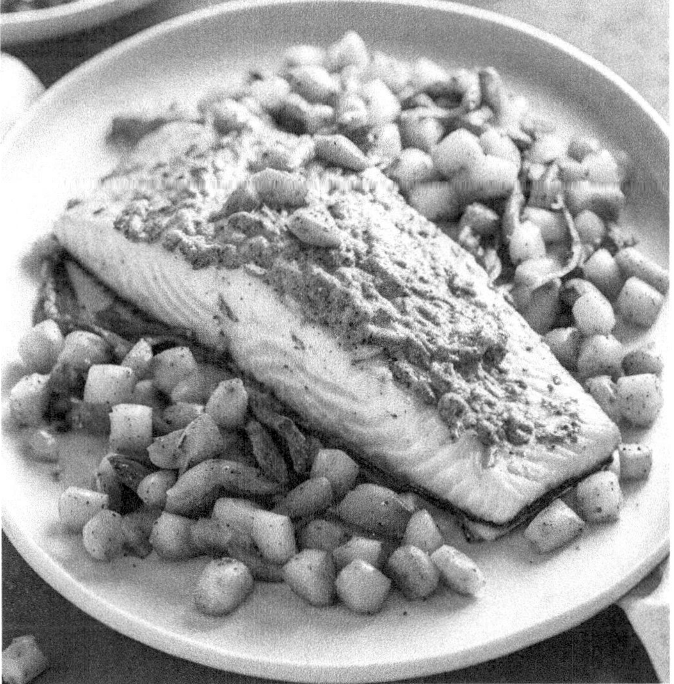

21. Parmesan Crusted Flounder

Ingredients:

- 4 flounder fillets (6 ounces each)
- 1/2 cup grated Parmesan cheese
- 1/4 cup whole grain breadcrumbs
- 2 tablespoons olive oil
- 2 cloves garlic, minced
- 1 tablespoon lemon juice
- 1 teaspoon dried basil

Instructions:

1. Preheat the oven to 400°F (200°C).
2. In a small bowl, mix the Parmesan cheese, breadcrumbs, olive oil, minced garlic, lemon juice, and dried basil.
3. Place the flounder fillets on a baking sheet lined with parchment paper.
4. Press the Parmesan mixture onto the top of each fillet.
5. Bake in the preheated oven for 12-15 minutes until the fish is cooked through and the crust is golden brown.
6. Serve hot.

Nutrition Info (per serving):

- Calories: 270
- Protein: 32g
- Carbohydrates: 5g
- Fiber: 1g
- Sugars: 1g
- Fat: 14g
- Saturated Fat: 3g

Serves: 4

Cooking Time: 15 minutes

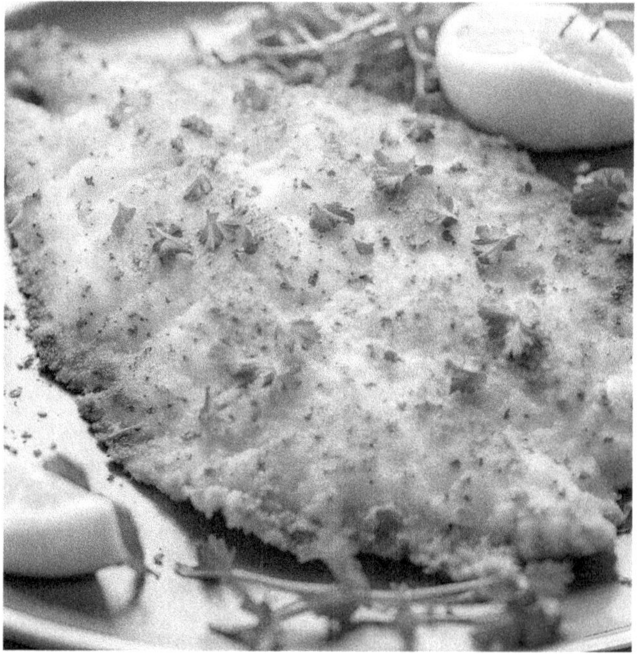

22. Broiled Tilapia with Tomato Caper Sauce

Ingredients:

- 4 tilapia fillets (6 ounces each)
- 2 tablespoons olive oil
- 1 teaspoon dried oregano
- 1 pint cherry tomatoes, halved
- 2 cloves garlic, minced
- 2 tablespoons capers, rinsed
- 1 tablespoon lemon juice
- 1/4 cup chopped fresh basil

Instructions:

1. Preheat the broiler on high.
2. Brush the tilapia fillets with 1 tablespoon of olive oil and sprinkle with dried oregano. Place them on a baking sheet lined with parchment paper.
3. Broil the tilapia for 4-5 minutes on each side until the fish is cooked through and flakes easily with a fork.
4. While the fish is broiling, heat the remaining olive oil in a skillet over medium heat.
5. Add the cherry tomatoes and garlic, cooking for 3-4 minutes until the tomatoes start to soften.
6. Stir in the capers and lemon juice, cooking for another 2 minutes.
7. Remove from heat and stir in the chopped fresh basil.
8. Spoon the tomato caper sauce over the broiled tilapia.
9. Serve hot.

Nutrition Info (per serving):

- Calories: 250
- Protein: 32g
- Carbohydrates: 6g
- Fiber: 2g
- Sugars: 3g
- Fat: 12g
- Saturated Fat: 2g

Serves: 4

Cooking Time: 20 minutes

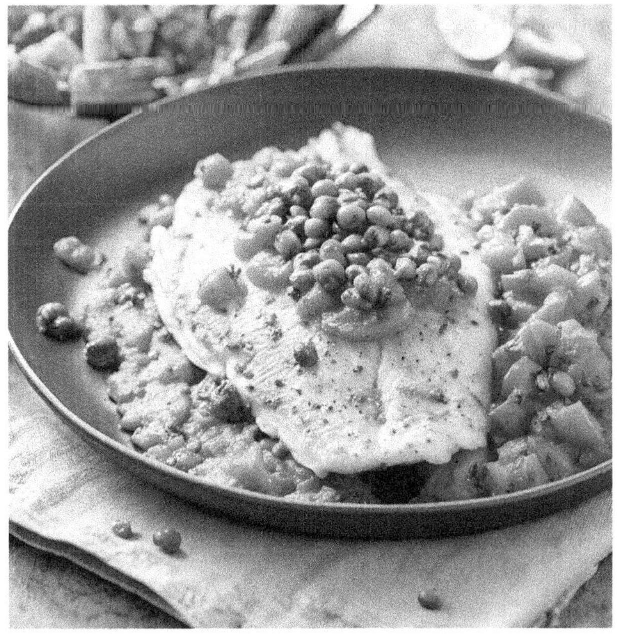

23. Scallop Ceviche

Ingredients:
- 1 pound large sea scallops, diced
- 1/2 cup freshly squeezed lime juice
- 1/4 cup freshly squeezed lemon juice
- 1/2 cup red onion, finely chopped
- 1 jalapeño, seeded and finely chopped
- 1/2 cup cilantro, chopped
- 1 avocado, diced
- 1/2 cup cherry tomatoes, quartered

Instructions:
1. In a large bowl, combine the diced scallops, lime juice, and lemon juice. Cover and refrigerate for 30 minutes, stirring occasionally until the scallops are opaque.
2. Add the red onion, jalapeño, and cilantro to the scallops. Mix well.
3. Gently fold in the diced avocado and cherry tomatoes.
4. Serve immediately.

Nutrition Info (per serving):
- Calories: 200
- Protein: 20g
- Carbohydrates: 10g
- Fiber: 4g
- Sugars: 3g
- Fat: 10g
- Saturated Fat: 1.5g

Serves: 4
Cooking Time: 40 minutes (including refrigeration)

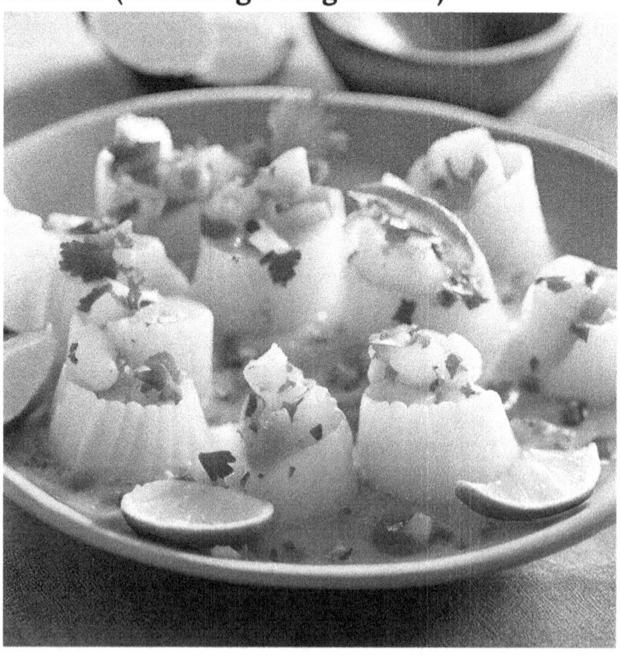

24. Fish Tacos with Lime Crema

Ingredients:

- 1 pound white fish fillets (such as tilapia or cod), cut into strips
- 2 tablespoons olive oil
- 1 teaspoon ground cumin
- 1 teaspoon paprika
- 8 small corn tortillas
- 2 cups shredded cabbage
- 1/2 cup grated carrots
- 1/4 cup chopped fresh cilantro

Lime Crema:

- 1/2 cup low-fat Greek yogurt
- 1 tablespoon lime juice
- 1 teaspoon lime zest

Instructions:

1. In a bowl, toss the fish strips with olive oil, ground cumin, and paprika.
2. Preheat a grill or grill pan to medium-high heat. Grill the fish strips for 2-3 minutes per side until cooked through.
3. In a small bowl, mix the Greek yogurt, lime juice, and lime zest to make the lime crema.
4. Warm the corn tortillas on the grill for about 30 seconds per side.
5. Assemble the tacos by placing grilled fish on the tortillas, topped with shredded cabbage, grated carrots, and chopped cilantro.
6. Drizzle with lime crema before serving.
7. Serve immediately.

Nutrition Info (per serving):

- Calories: 280
- Protein: 24g
- Carbohydrates: 24g
- Fiber: 5g
- Sugars: 3g
- Fat: 10g
- Saturated Fat: 2g

Serves: 4

Cooking Time: 20 minutes

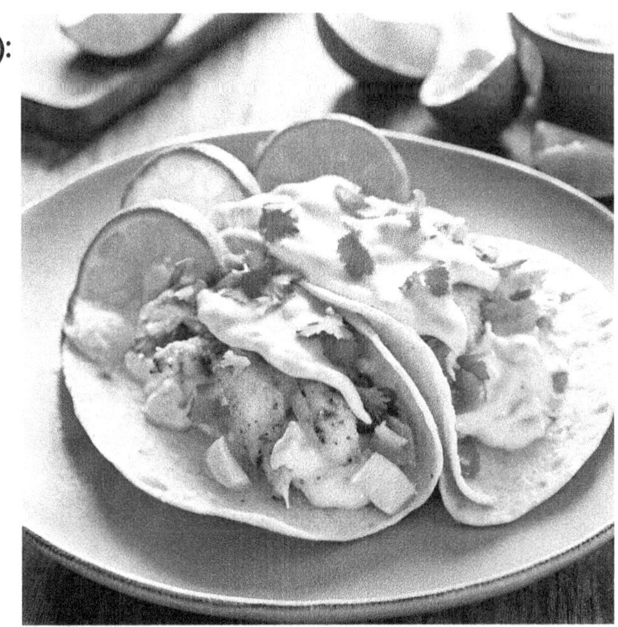

25. Seafood Frittata

Ingredients:

- 8 large eggs
- 1/4 cup low-fat milk
- 1/2 cup grated Parmesan cheese
- 1/2 pound shrimp, peeled and deveined
- 1/2 pound crabmeat
- 1 cup spinach, chopped
- 1/2 cup cherry tomatoes, halved
- 1 tablespoon olive oil
- 2 cloves garlic, minced
- 1 teaspoon dried oregano

Instructions:

1. Preheat the oven to 375°F (190°C).
2. In a large bowl, whisk the eggs, milk, and Parmesan cheese.
3. Heat the olive oil in an oven-safe skillet over medium heat. Add the minced garlic and cook for 1 minute until fragrant.
4. Add the shrimp and cook for 2-3 minutes until pink. Add the crabmeat, chopped spinach, cherry tomatoes, and dried oregano. Cook for another 2-3 minutes.
5. Pour the egg mixture into the skillet, stirring gently to combine.
6. Transfer the skillet to the preheated oven and bake for 15-20 minutes until the frittata is set and golden brown.
7. Serve hot.

Nutrition Info (per serving):

- Calories: 250
- Protein: 28g
- Carbohydrates: 6g
- Fiber: 1g
- Sugars: 2g
- Fat: 12g
- Saturated Fat: 3g

Serves: 4

Cooking Time: 25 minutes

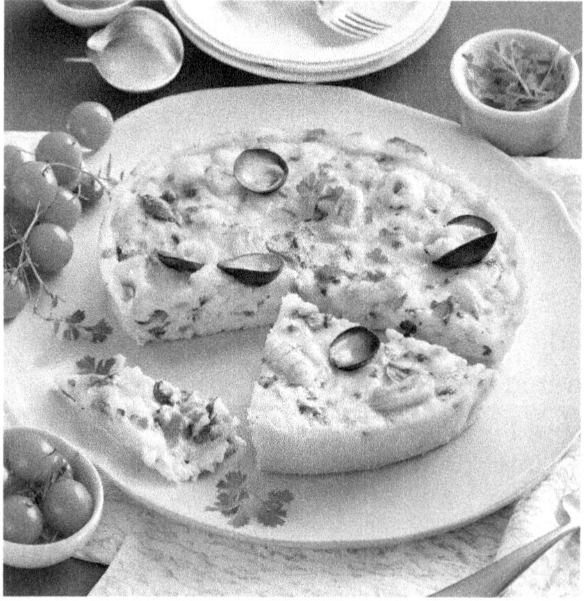

26. Sea Bass with Mango Salsa

Ingredients:

- 4 sea bass fillets (6 ounces each)
- 2 tablespoons olive oil
- 1 tablespoon lemon juice
- 1 teaspoon dried thyme

Mango Salsa:

- 1 ripe mango, diced
- 1/4 cup red bell pepper, finely chopped
- 1/4 cup red onion, finely chopped
- 1 jalapeño, seeded and finely chopped
- 1/4 cup cilantro, chopped
- 1 tablespoon lime juice

Instructions:

1. Preheat the oven to 375°F (190°C).
2. In a small bowl, mix the olive oil, lemon juice, and dried thyme.
3. Brush the mixture over the sea bass fillets.
4. Place the fillets on a baking sheet lined with parchment paper and bake for 15-20 minutes until the fish is cooked through and flakes easily with a fork.
5. In a medium bowl, combine the diced mango, red bell pepper, red onion, jalapeño, cilantro, and lime juice to make the mango salsa.
6. Serve the sea bass fillets topped with mango salsa.
7. Serve hot.

Nutrition Info (per serving):

- Calories: 310
- Protein: 32g
- Carbohydrates: 10g
- Fiber: 2g
- Sugars: 7g
- Fat: 16g
- Saturated Fat: 3g

Serves: 4
Cooking Time: 25 minutes

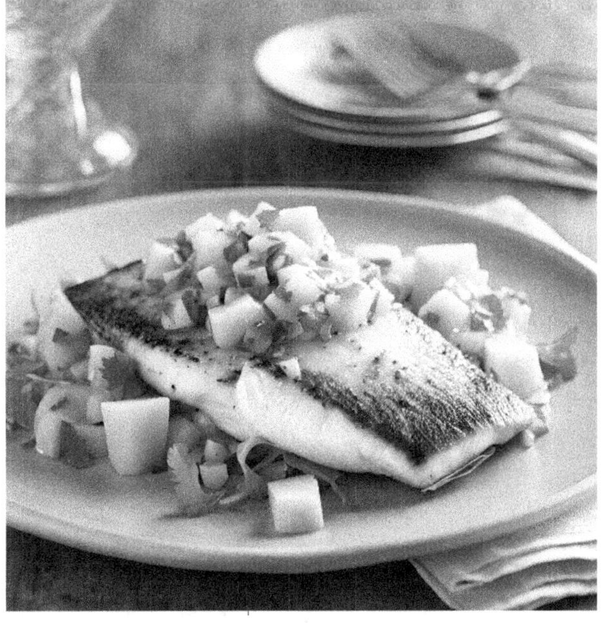

27. Shrimp and Grits

Ingredients:

- 1 pound shrimp, peeled and deveined
- 1 tablespoon olive oil
- 2 cloves garlic, minced
- 1 cup stone-ground grits
- 4 cups low-sodium chicken broth
- 1/2 cup low-fat milk
- 1/4 cup grated Parmesan cheese
- 1 tablespoon lemon juice
- 1/4 cup chopped green onions

Instructions:

1. In a medium saucepan, bring the chicken broth to a boil. Slowly whisk in the grits.
2. Reduce heat to low and cook the grits, stirring occasionally, for about 20-25 minutes until thickened.
3. Stir in the milk and Parmesan cheese until creamy. Remove from heat and cover to keep warm.
4. In a large skillet, heat the olive oil over medium heat. Add the minced garlic and cook for 1 minute until fragrant.
5. Add the shrimp and cook for 2-3 minutes on each side until pink and cooked through.
6. Stir in the lemon juice and chopped green onions.
7. Serve the shrimp over the creamy grits.
8. Serve hot.

Nutrition Info (per serving):

- Calories: 320
- Protein: 28g
- Carbohydrates: 30g
- Fiber: 2g
- Sugars: 3g
- Fat: 12g
- Saturated Fat: 3g

Serves: 4

Cooking Time: 30 minutes

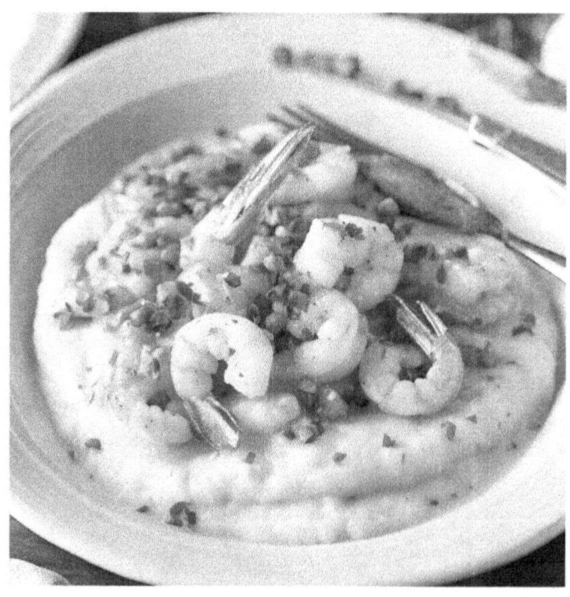

10-WEEK MEAL PLAN

Week 1
Monday
- Breakfast: Almond Flour Pancakes
- Lunch: Chicken and Asparagus Lemon Stir Fry
- Dinner: Grilled Salmon with Dill and Lemon

Tuesday
- Breakfast: Blueberry Spinach Smoothie
- Lunch: Vegetable Lasagna
- Dinner: Baked Cod with Cherry Tomatoes

Wednesday
- Breakfast: Cottage Cheese Pancakes
- Lunch: Mediterranean Turkey Meatloaf
- Dinner: Seafood Gumbo

Thursday
- Breakfast: Oat Flour Waffles
- Lunch: Spinach and Mushroom Soup
- Dinner: Pesto Baked Salmon

Friday
- Breakfast: Chia and Coconut Rice Pudding
- Lunch: Turkey and Sweet Potato Skillet
- Dinner: Seared Tuna Steaks

Saturday
- Breakfast: Breakfast Salad
- Lunch: Eggplant and Chickpea Stew
- Dinner: Fisherman's Stew

Sunday
- Breakfast: Sweet Potato Bowl
- Lunch: Zucchini Basil Soup
- Dinner: Swordfish Steaks with Cilantro Lime Butter

Week 2
Monday
- Breakfast: Avocado Green Smoothie
- Lunch: Baked Tomatoes with Pesto
- Dinner: Herb-Crusted Tilapia

Tuesday
- Breakfast: Ricotta & Fig Toast
- Lunch: Moroccan Chicken Tagine
- Dinner: Broiled Scallops with Parmesan Crust

Wednesday
- Breakfast: Pumpkin Seed Granola
- Lunch: Stuffed Portobello Mushrooms
- Dinner: Shrimp Risotto

Thursday
- Breakfast: Congee
- Lunch: Chicken Paillard
- Dinner: Barbecue Glazed Salmon

Friday
- Breakfast: Millet Pudding
- Lunch: Carrot and Apple Slaw
- Dinner: Grilled Shrimp Skewers

Saturday
- Breakfast: Mushroom & Spinach Toast
- Lunch: Turkey Vegetable Stir-Fry
- Dinner: Miso Glazed Cod

Sunday
- Breakfast: Soy Yogurt with Granola
- Lunch: Zucchini and Tomato Stew
- Dinner: Sea Bass with Mango Salsa

Week 3

Monday
- Breakfast: Banana Pancakes
- Lunch: Chicken Soup with Vegetables
- Dinner: Vietnamese Fish Tacos

Tuesday
- Breakfast: Baked Pears with Walnuts
- Lunch: Broccoli Salad
- Dinner: Scallop Ceviche

Wednesday
- Breakfast: Bell Pepper and Tofu Stir-Fry
- Lunch: Asian Cabbage Salad
- Dinner: Chicken and Broccoli Alfredo

Thursday
- Breakfast: Grilled Asparagus with Lemon
- Lunch: Eggplant and Tomato Stir-Fry
- Dinner: Parmesan Crusted Flounder

Friday
- Breakfast: Zucchini Noodles with Pesto
- Lunch: Kale and Quinoa Salad
- Dinner: Chicken Fajitas

Saturday
- Breakfast: Millet Pudding
- Lunch: Stuffed Portobello Mushrooms
- Dinner: Shrimp and Grits

Sunday
- Breakfast: Sweet Corn and Zucchini Fritters
- Lunch: Spinach and White Bean Soup
- Dinner: Turkey and Quinoa Stuffed Peppers

Week 4

Monday
- Breakfast: Sweet Potato Bowl
- Lunch: Tomato Basil Soup
- Dinner: Chicken Cacciatore

Tuesday
- Breakfast: Ricotta & Fig Toast
- Lunch: Moroccan Vegetable Tagine
- Dinner: Broiled Tilapia with Tomato Caper Sauce

Wednesday
- Breakfast: Millet Pudding
- Lunch: Carrot and Apple Slaw
- Dinner: Mediterranean Fish Soup

Thursday
- Breakfast: Mushroom & Spinach Toast
- Lunch: Chicken Paillard
- Dinner: Seafood Frittata

Friday
- Breakfast: Soy Yogurt with Granola
- Lunch: Zucchini and Tomato Stew
- Dinner: Sea Bass with Mango Salsa

Saturday
- Breakfast: Avocado Green Smoothie
- Lunch: Baked Tomatoes with Pesto
- Dinner: Grilled Salmon with Dill and Lemon

Sunday
- Breakfast: Blueberry Spinach Smoothie
- Lunch: Vegetable Lasagna
- Dinner: Seared Tuna Steaks

Week 5

Monday
- Breakfast: Pumpkin Seed Granola
- Lunch: Spinach and Mushroom Soup
- Dinner: Swordfish Steaks with Cilantro Lime Butter

Tuesday
- Breakfast: Congee
- Lunch: Eggplant and Chickpea Stew
- Dinner: Pesto Baked Salmon

Wednesday
- Breakfast: Banana Pancakes
- Lunch: Mediterranean Turkey Meatloaf
- Dinner: Fisherman's Stew

Thursday
- Breakfast: Baked Pears with Walnuts
- Lunch: Carrot and Apple Slaw
- Dinner: Chicken Fajitas

Friday
- Breakfast: Mushroom & Spinach Toast
- Lunch: Bell Pepper and Tofu Stir-Fry
- Dinner: Barbecue Glazed Salmon

Saturday
- Breakfast: Millet Pudding
- Lunch: Asian Cabbage Salad
- Dinner: Miso Glazed Cod

Sunday
- Breakfast: Sweet Corn and Zucchini Fritters
- Lunch: Zucchini and Tomato Stew
- Dinner: Parmesan Crusted Flounder

Week 6

Monday
- Breakfast: Buckwheat Waffles
- Lunch: Chicken Ratatouille
- Dinner: Tuna Salad Stuffed Tomatoes

Tuesday
- Breakfast: Cucumber and Hummus Plate
- Lunch: Garlic Spinach Sauté
- Dinner: Herb-Roasted Chicken Breast

Wednesday
- Breakfast: Bell Pepper and Tofu Stir-Fry
- Lunch: Asian Tofu and Vegetable Stew
- Dinner: Salmon and Pea Tagliatelle

Thursday
- Breakfast: Millet Pudding
- Lunch: Moroccan Chicken Tagine
- Dinner: Szechuan Chicken Stir Fry

Friday
- Breakfast: Grilled Asparagus with Lemon
- Lunch: Tomato Basil Soup
- Dinner: Grilled Shrimp Skewers

Saturday
- Breakfast: Zucchini Noodles with Pesto
- Lunch: Sweet Potato and Lentil Soup
- Dinner: Vietnamese Fish Tacos

Sunday
- Breakfast: Bell Pepper and Tofu Stir-Fry
- Lunch: Eggplant and Tomato Stir-Fry
- Dinner: Scallop Ceviche

Week 7

Monday
- Breakfast: Banana Pancakes
- Lunch: Chicken and Broccoli Alfredo
- Dinner: Broiled Tilapia with Tomato Caper Sauce

Tuesday
- Breakfast: Avocado Green Smoothie
- Lunch: Kale and White Bean Stew
- Dinner: Sea Bass with Mango Salsa

Wednesday
- Breakfast: Soy Yogurt with Granola
- Lunch: Spinach and Mushroom Soup
- Dinner: Shrimp Risotto

Thursday
- Breakfast: Sweet Corn and Zucchini Fritters
- Lunch: Moroccan Vegetable Tagine
- Dinner: Chicken Cacciatore

Friday
- Breakfast: Millet Pudding
- Lunch: Baked Tomatoes with Pesto
- Dinner: Parmesan Crusted Flounder

Saturday
- Breakfast: Ricotta & Fig Toast
- Lunch: Chicken Soup with Vegetables
- Dinner: Broiled Scallops with Parmesan Crust

Sunday
- Breakfast: Pumpkin Seed Granola
- Lunch: Eggplant and Chickpea Stew
- Dinner: Fisherman's Stew

Week 8

Monday
- Breakfast: Congee
- Lunch: Carrot and Apple Slaw
- Dinner: Mediterranean Fish Soup

Tuesday
- Breakfast: Mushroom & Spinach Toast
- Lunch: Zucchini and Tomato Stew
- Dinner: Barbecue Glazed Salmon

Wednesday
- Breakfast: Millet Pudding
- Lunch: Bell Pepper and Tofu Stir-Fry
- Dinner: Swordfish Steaks with Cilantro Lime Butter

Thursday
- Breakfast: Grilled Asparagus with Lemon
- Lunch: Spinach and White Bean Soup
- Dinner: Herb-Crusted Tilapia

Friday
- Breakfast: Zucchini Noodles with Pesto
- Lunch: Sweet Potato and Lentil Soup
- Dinner: Seared Tuna Steaks

Saturday
- Breakfast: Avocado Green Smoothie
- Lunch: Chicken and Broccoli Alfredo
- Dinner: Tuna Salad Stuffed Tomatoes

Sunday
- Breakfast: Bell Pepper and Tofu Stir-Fry
- Lunch: Chicken Ratatouille
- Dinner: Shrimp and Grits

Week 9

Monday
- Breakfast: Banana Pancakes
- Lunch: Moroccan Chicken Tagine
- Dinner: Vietnamese Fish Tacos

Tuesday
- Breakfast: Soy Yogurt with Granola
- Lunch: Tomato Basil Soup
- Dinner: Pesto Baked Salmon

Wednesday
- Breakfast: Pumpkin Seed Granola
- Lunch: Sweet Potato and Lentil Soup
- Dinner: Shrimp Risotto

Thursday
- Breakfast: Ricotta & Fig Toast
- Lunch: Kale and White Bean Stew
- Dinner: Chicken Cacciatore

Friday
- Breakfast: Congee
- Lunch: Spinach and Mushroom Soup
- Dinner: Broiled Tilapia with Tomato Caper Sauce

Saturday
- Breakfast: Mushroom & Spinach Toast
- Lunch: Chicken Soup with Vegetables
- Dinner: Broiled Scallops with Parmesan Crust

Sunday
- Breakfast: Millet Pudding
- Lunch: Baked Tomatoes with Pesto
- Dinner: Fisherman's Stew

Week 10

Monday
- Breakfast: Grilled Asparagus with Lemon
- Lunch: Zucchini and Tomato Stew
- Dinner: Parmesan Crusted Flounder

Tuesday
- Breakfast: Zucchini Noodles with Pesto
- Lunch: Eggplant and Chickpea Stew
- Dinner: Scallop Ceviche

Wednesday
- Breakfast: Avocado Green Smoothie
- Lunch: Carrot and Apple Slaw
- Dinner: Salmon and Pea Tagliatelle

Thursday
- Breakfast: Pumpkin Seed Granola
- Lunch: Bell Pepper and Tofu Stir-Fry
- Dinner: Swordfish Steaks with Cilantro Lime Butter

Friday
- Breakfast: Ricotta & Fig Toast
- Lunch: Chicken Ratatouille
- Dinner: Shrimp and Grits

Saturday
- Breakfast: Congee
- Lunch: Moroccan Vegetable Tagine
- Dinner: Mediterranean Fish Soup

Sunday
- Breakfast: Mushroom & Spinach Toast
- Lunch: Spinach and White Bean Soup
- Dinner: Barbecue Glazed Salmon

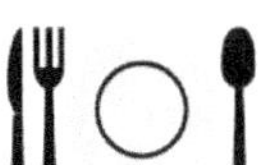

Weekly Meal planner+ Journal

	BREAKFAST	LUNCH	DINNER	SNACKS
MON				
TUE				
WED				
THU				
FRI				
SAT				
SUN				

What are your main goals for following the Melanoma Diet? Reflect on both short-term and long-term goals related to your health and well-being.

Weekly Meal planner+ Journal

	BREAKFAST	LUNCH	DINNER	SNACKS
MON				
TUE				
WED				
THU				
FRI				
SAT				
SUN				

How do you currently feel about your diet and its impact on your health? Consider your current eating habits and how they make you feel physically and emotionally.

Weekly Meal planner+ Journal

	BREAKFAST	LUNCH	DINNER	SNACKS
MON				
TUE				
WED				
THU				
FRI				
SAT				
SUN				

What challenges do you anticipate facing when changing your diet? Identify potential obstacles that might arise and think about how you can address them.

Weekly Meal planner+ Journal

	BREAKFAST	LUNCH	DINNER	SNACKS
MON				
TUE				
WED				
THU				
FRI				
SAT				
SUN				

Are there any foods you are currently eating that you suspect might not be beneficial for your condition?
Reflect on any dietary choices that may need to be reduced or eliminated.

Weekly Meal planner+ Journal

	BREAKFAST	LUNCH	DINNER	SNACKS
MON				
TUE				
WED				
THU				
FRI				
SAT				
SUN				

How do you plan to incorporate more fresh fruits and vegetables into your meals? Brainstorm practical ways to increase your intake of nutrient-rich produce.

....

....

....

....

....

....

Weekly Meal planner+ Journal

	BREAKFAST	LUNCH	DINNER	SNACKS
MON				
TUE				
WED				
THU				
FRI				
SAT				
SUN				

How will you prepare yourself for dining out or social events while following this diet? Consider how you can make healthy choices when eating outside of your home.

....

....

....

....

....

....

Weekly Meal planner+ Journal

	BREAKFAST	LUNCH	DINNER	SNACKS
MON				
TUE				
WED				
THU				
FRI				
SAT				
SUN				

What support systems do you have in place to help you maintain your dietary changes? Identify friends, family, or support groups that can offer encouragement and assistance.

Weekly Meal planner+ Journal

	BREAKFAST	LUNCH	DINNER	SNACKS
MON				
TUE				
WED				
THU				
FRI				
SAT				
SUN				

What new recipes or cooking techniques are you excited to try? List some healthy recipes or cooking methods you want to explore.

Scan the QR code below to get a surprise bonus!